DISPENSING OP̶T̶I̶C̶S̶

DISPENSING OPTICS

Ajay Kumar Bhootra
B Optom DOS FAO FOAI FCLI
ICLEP FIACLE (Australia)
Diploma in Sportvision (UK)
CEO and Dean
Krishnalaya School of Optometry
Kolkata, West Bengal, India

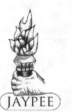

JAYPEE *The Health Sciences Publisher*

New Delhi | London | Philadelphia | Panama

Jaypee Brothers Medical Publishers (P) Ltd

Headquarters

Jaypee Brothers Medical Publishers (P) Ltd
4838/24, Ansari Road, Daryaganj
New Delhi 110 002, India
Phone: +91-11-43574357
Fax: +91-11-43574314
Email: jaypee@jaypeebrothers.com

Overseas Offices

J.P. Medical Ltd
83 Victoria Street, London
SW1H 0HW (UK)
Phone: +44 20 3170 8910
Fax: +44 (0)20 3008 6180
Email: info@jpmedpub.com

Jaypee Medical Inc
The Bourse
111 South Independence Mall East
Suite 835, Philadelphia, PA 19106, USA
Phone: +1 267-519-9789
Email: jpmed.us@gmail.com

Jaypee Brothers Medical Publishers (P) Ltd
Bhotahity, Kathmandu, Nepal
Phone: +977-9741283608
Email: kathmandu@jaypeebrothers.com

Jaypee-Highlights Medical Publishers Inc
City of Knowledge, Bld. 237, Clayton
Panama City, Panama
Phone: +1 507-301-0496
Fax: +1 507-301-0499
Email: cservice@jphmedical.com

Jaypee Brothers Medical Publishers (P) Ltd
17/1-B Babar Road, Block-B, Shaymali
Mohammadpur, Dhaka-1207
Bangladesh
Mobile: +08801912003485
Email: jaypeedhaka@gmail.com

Website: www.jaypeebrothers.com
Website: www.jaypeedigital.com

Dispensing Optics

First Edition: **2016**

ISBN 978-93-5250-013-0

Printed at Rajkamal Electric Press, Plot No. 2, Phase-IV, Kundli, Haryana.

Free computerized eye examination by qualified optometrists
Pay for your glasses—get your spouse glasses free
Exchange your old spectacle for the brand new one
Buy one, get one free

If you look at lots of such communications that talk about the way an optician releases their media statements, I wonder most people would get the message that opticians are also motivated by sheer driving force of sales. Well, this is justified to achieve the business objective but is never enough to bring the sense of accomplishment that a dispensing optician realizes through the healthcare approach. A patient does not go to an optician just because the products he sells, he goes to him because he believes that the optician would help him selecting an appropriate frame and advice suitable lens to match his visual needs. This is a real challenge for the opticians to develop near equal expertise of healthcare provider. More so because no formal training facility is available for optical dispensing that can form the basic foundation for complete success. I do not know how people in the industry think, but I had my own experience and I feel mastering the basic skills of the art builds high level of confidence and help you establish your creditability to develop your practice as a successful dispensing optician. I remember my first preceptor, Late Sri SM Bose. "No way," I could forget him; he did a bit of foundation that is still rolling off my tongue effortlessly. Today, it is hard to shut me up when it comes to dispensing optics. Perhaps that is enough to show how much I am obsessed. To me, the art of optical dispensing is like an art of composing new melodies. When you sculpt the spectacle to fit on the wearer's face, your hand moves like the notes of the melody. The final fit that snugly holds the spectacle frame on the face is like a perfect sound that pleases the wearer's and allows him to enjoy the eyewear with ease of use.

The success in optical dispensing needs a unique blend of technical skills, soft skills and observation power with extreme level of judgmental excellence. You need to invest your time and energy to train yourself to learn the basic science of ophthalmic optics, develop technical skills and necessary soft skills to excel in the art. What I mean to state is that there is more than one reason for training and skill development program in the optical dispensing. But there are not much of the resource materials available. That is probably one of the biggest driving factors that prompted me to compile all my experiences in this fascinating book that I named as *Dispensing Optics*.

Dispensing Optics is filled with theoretical and practical information about the art and science of the spectacle dispensing. You will find this book absolutely reader friendly. At the start of each chapter, there is an outline that gives you a fair deal of idea about the objectives of the chapter; and at the end the chapter, the important take-away learnings are summarized as Points to Remember to ensure that you do not miss anything before you move forward. Read the book with your eyes, peeled for the main idea. Dip in and out of it on an ongoing basis and you will find your dispensing skills improving day by day.

I am very much enthusiastic about this exciting work and it gets to me when I see the simplicity of the book. Most contents of the book are compiled from the knowledge that I have gathered from the training programs I have attended and my practical experiences. If you take the techniques found in this book and apply them, I promise you that you will be more successful than most other. A bold promise for sure, but I expect nothing less than best for you. You will also get me as your personal coach, giving you free tips throughout the year on my website:

www.specsguru.co.in

A word of advice—while you read, immerse yourself in the book and practice what is being explained. You must absorb what is being said. Read the book from beginning to end. Do not skip any chapter. Once you have done that, you can then refer back to individual chapter to sharpen your skills. Please enjoy the book as much as I enjoyed bringing it to you.

Ajay Kumar Bhootra

ACKNOWLEDGMENTS

As far as I understand, no creation in this world is a solo effort. Neither is this book. I have received enormous inputs of several persons from the time I conceived the idea of this book to its present shape. I would like to acknowledge everybody's effort and would like to thank all of them for bringing it to this shape. Special thanks to:

- My readers and students, for their support and love.
- God, who cares for me.
- My amazing list of patients and clients, because of whom I could have so varied experience.
- All my trainers and coaches, who had been instrumental in providing me training on different occasions.
- My friends and family members.
- And all the people I met during my working experience and training, who helped me understand my subject.
- Above all, the members of my organization Himalaya Optical.

I am fond of reading books on various subjects. That is why, while reading this book, you may notice that the contents of this book are influenced by many books. Probably, that makes the disk rolls in favor of the book.

I am also one of the biggest admirers of Mr Darryl Meister who has been an active member of the Optical Industry and is one of the authorities in the field of ophthalmic optics. His articles published in magazines such as Optical World, Clinical and Experimental Optometry, Lens Talk and Refractive Eye Care Management, have been a great source of information for me while working with this book.

And, finally, I would like to recollect my old memories when I had my mentor Late Sri KK Binani whom I miss so much even now.

CONTENTS

CHAPTER 1

INTRODUCTION TO DISPENSING OPTICS

The optical dispensing provides huge scope for manifestations of emotional dimensions by changing the way we see. Most theories and practices of dispensing optics are based on the basic principles of ophthalmic optics. The purpose of this chapter is to set the context with the relevant topics of ophthalmic optics and acquaint the reader with the basic principles and terminology essential to establish profound understanding of the subject.

Dispensing optics is the science of dispensing eyeglasses and contact lenses based on the prescription of an eye care practitioner. The eye care practitioner prescribes a lens power based upon which the dispensing optician dispenses the correct spectacle lens. Most theories of dispensing optics follow the principles of geometrical optics. The principles of geometrical optics are based on the assumption that light rays always travel in straight lines and in a given direction when they are in free space but change their direction, when they encounter any matter.

Laws of reflection and laws of refraction are two main theories of geometrical optics. It also follows some of the principles of wave optics. Wave optics assumes that light travels in waves. Interference, diffraction and polarization are three main principles of wave optics. Interference is the ability of the light wave to interfere with itself. Diffraction is the ability of the light wave to spread after passing through an aperture. Polarization refers to the phenomenon in which waves of light are restricted to a given direction of vibration. Light rays after transmitting through the various ocular structures fall on the retina where the stimuli for vision is formed that produces four types of visual perceptions—light sense, form sense, color sense and sense of contrast. The pathway behind the retina carries the signal to the visual cortex where all information is integrated into one single visual perception.

Optical dispensing is also an art—that teaches how to make the spectacle and sculpt the spectacle frame so that it makes contact with patient's face comfortably, looks good and also serves the desired function. The art can be learned and mastered by practice and experience. Sculpting the spectacle frame to fit the patient's face needs skillful hands because both anthropometric and cosmetic demands are to be met. The process of dispensing starts right from selecting a frame to taking measurements and fitting the eyewear on the patient's face. Discovery of truths from the patients and discloser of truths to the patients are also two important building blocks of the art.

Today optical dispensing is considered to be an important part of holistic eye care. The reasons are fairly simple. Even the best refraction may not provide the desired results if the lenses are not dispensed effectively. Lenses are used to maximize the vision and lenses are also used to maintain the vision. This implies that enhancement and maintenance are two important goals of optical dispensing. A rightly selected lens material coupled with appropriate lens design is critical to achieve the desired goals; and this is very important aspect of holistic eye care that also comes within the scope of dispensing optics.

LIGHT

Visible light is a small part of electromagnetic spectrum (Fig. 1.1) ranging from 380 nm to 760 nm that lies between ultraviolet (UV) and infrared (IR) portions with UV rays lying at shorter wavelength end and IR rays lying next to longer wavelength end. Light rays are able to travel through a vacuum or a medium. Light travels very rapidly. In vacuum, the speed of light is 186,282 m/s or nearly 300,000 km/s. Wavelength, frequency and energy describe the properties of light. Wavelength of light is the distance from one peak to the next. It is measured in nanometer or micrometer or angstrom. Our eyes interpret these wavelengths as different colors. If only a limited range of wavelengths enter our eyes, we interpret as certain color. If all wavelengths of visible light enter, we interpret them as white light. If no wavelengths in the visible range are present, we interpret as dark. Human eyes are most sensitive to yellow color which has the wavelength ranging from 570 to 590 nm. Red color is the longest wavelength of light and violet color is the shortest wavelength of light that the human eye can see. Frequency is the number of times per second that a wave vibrates up and down. The longer wavelengths will vibrate fewer times in a given time interval than the shorter ones. Frequency is measured in hertz. Longer wavelength has lower frequency and the shorter wavelength has higher frequency.

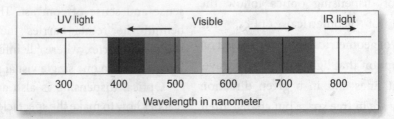

FIGURE 1.1: Electromagnetic spectrum

Red color has the lowest frequency. Both wavelength and frequency are of high importance in determining the speed or velocity of light. We can also characterize light by the energy that it carries. Shorter wavelength of light carries intense energy than longer wavelength of light. They carry enough energy with them to damage ocular structure. Classically, the danger of X-rays and gamma rays at the shorter wavelength end is well-known. Shorter wavelength of violet and blue light also spread within the globe and thereby creates veiling effect that affects the sense of contrast.

OPHTHALMIC LENSES

Ophthalmic lenses are transparent bodies that bend light by virtue of the curvature of their surfaces. A surface is formed when a given curve is revolved around a given axis. In case of a spherical lens the surface is formed by rotating a circle about any diameter. A plane surface has zero curvature and may be considered as a spherical surface with infinite radius. A cylinder surface is generated by rotating a straight line about another straight line that is parallel to it. A toric surface is generated by rotating a surface of revolution of a circle around an axis which is outside the circle. Aspheric curves are obtained by rotating a straight line around another line that intersects a conicoid solid, i.e. around axis of symmetry of conicoid solid. The curvature of a surface is given by the angle through which the surface turns in a unit length of arc. The curvature determines how steep or flat the lens surface is. The curvature is specified as inversely proportional to the radius. It implies that the large radius of curvature will have flatter lens surface and curvature will have flatter lens surface and

smaller radius of curvature will have steeper lens surface.

Plus lenses are the combination of prisms base to base while minus lenses are the combination of prisms apex to apex. Understanding spectacle lenses as a combination of prisms is the key to understand how lenses direct light and correct vision. The image viewed through a prism always moves towards the apex, it implies that plus lenses will show "up motion" when it is taken down as the apex of prism lies at the top edge; "towards right" when the lens is taken to left as the apex of prism lies at the right edge and so on. Minus lens will show "down motion" if the lens is taken down as the apex of the prism lies at the center of the lens and so on as shown in Figure 1.2.

Light traveling from air to a prism always bends towards its base. Since a plus lens is the combination of prisms that lies base to base, light rays traveling from air to prism will bend towards its base. It implies that all lights passing through a plus or convex lens will converge to a point as shown in the Figure 1.3. A minus lens is a combination of prism that lies apex to apex. Light rays traveling from air to prism will bend towards its base. It implies that all lights passing through a minus or concave lens will diverge. The optical center of the lens is the singular point through which light rays pass without being deviated.

All ophthalmic lenses have two principal meridians. A meridian is an imaginary line that passes through the optical center of the lens as shown in Figure 1.4. A lens has many meridians, but there are two principal

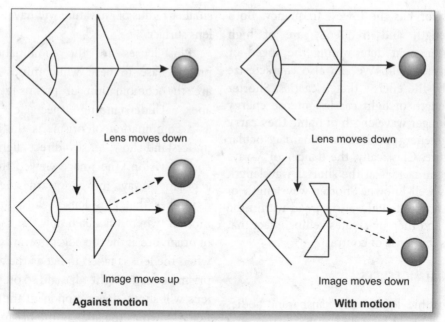

FIGURE 1.2: Movement observed through plus and minus lenses

meridians those lie perpendicular to each other and meet at the optical center of the lens. The rays of light passing through this meeting point travel undeviated. When these two meridians carry same power, the lens is known as spherical lens and when these two meridians carry different power, the lens is known as sphero-cylinder lens.

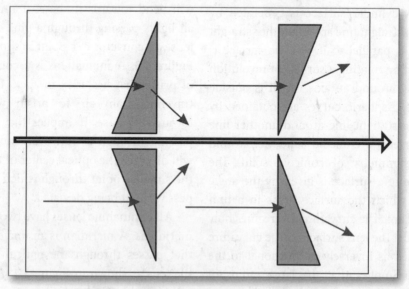

FIGURE 1.3: Light rays passing through Cx and CC lens

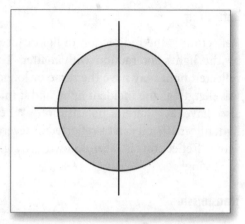

FIGURE 1.4: Two principal meridians of a lens

cross that shows the dioptric strength of the lens along the respective meridian. Both the principal meridians are perpendicular to each other as shown in Figure 1.5, e.g. if one principal meridian is at 90°, other would be at 180° and so on. The point at which the two principal meridians meet is known as optical center of the lens. Rays of light passing through this point goes without any deviation as there is no effect of prism at this point. A hypothetical straight line that connects the center of curvature of each lens surface is known as optical axis. The two principal meridians are commonly known as axis meridian and power meridian. Axis meridian has the minimum lens power and power meridian has the maximum lens power as shown in the Table 1.1.

In case of plano-cylinder lens, one meridian has no power and other carries the lens power.

The two principal meridians of an ophthalmic lens are represented diagrammatically in the form of an optical

Table 1.1:

Lens power in axis meridian and power meridian		
Lens power	*Axis meridian*	*Power meridian*
Spherical	Amount of spherical	Same as axis meridian
Plano-cylinder	Plano	Cylinder element
Sphero-cylinder	Spherical element	Summation of both spherical and cylinder

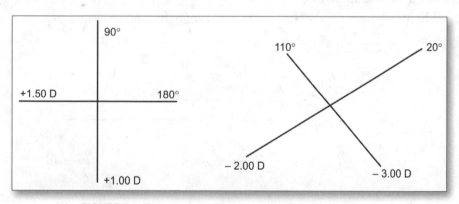

FIGURE 1.5: Optical cross with principal meridians at given axis

INTERACTIONS OF LIGHT WITH OPHTHALMIC LENSES

When light travels through a medium it is influenced by the physical, chemical and other properties of the matter. This is called interaction of light. The interactions occur in the form of emission, absorption, transmission and reflection. This interaction determines the appearance of everything we see. Different matters respond to light differently. Transparent matters transmit more light and absorb less whereas translucent matters absorb more light and transmit less. Opaque matters absorb most light. Ophthalmic lenses are transparent bodies and when light interacts with ophthalmic lenses three phenomenon occur as shown in Flowchart 1.1.

Absorption

When the spectrum of the light passes through a medium, it appears to have lost certain wavelength. This is because of light absorption. Selective absorption is the basis for objects having color. A red apple appears as red because it absorbs other colors of the visible spectrum and reflects only red light.

Reflection

Reflection is the redirection of light caused by the light's interaction with matter. The reflected light may have the same or longer wavelength as the incident light, and it may also have a different polarization. When light hits matter, it can be reflected in several ways. Reflection is also known as light scattering.

Transmission

When light interferes with transparent medium, refraction occurs and light is transmitted. Ophthalmic lenses allow us to see because of light transmission through them.

SIGN CONVENTIONS

Sign conventions used to denote ophthalmic lenses is based upon the direction of light. It is being assumed that light always travels from left to right in straight line.

The conventions used are:
1. All dimensions are measured from the vertex of the lens to the point in question, or image point.
2. Any measurement taken in the course of light is taken as positive and the measurement taken against the course of light is taken as negative.

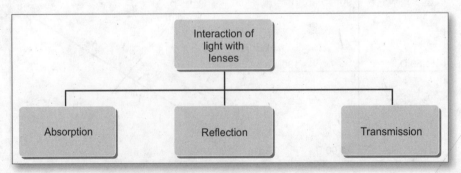

FLOWCHART 1.1: Interaction of light with lenses

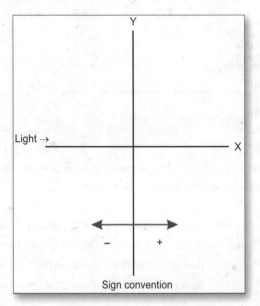

FIGURE 1.6: Sign convention

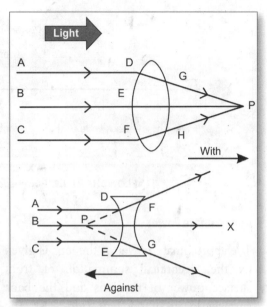

FIGURE 1.7: Convex and concave lens

Look at the Figure 1.6 in which distance measured to the left of X axis is negative, distance measured to the right of the X axis is positive, distances above the optical axis are positive and distances below the optical axis are negative.

The light rays emanating from an object point and passing through a convex lens has a principal focus in front of the lens and the focal length measured from the lens surface to image point is with the direction of light travel, hence it is taken to be "+". The light rays emanating from an object point and passing through a concave lens has a principal focus behind the lens and the focal length measured from the lens to image point is against the direction of light travel, hence it is taken to be "—" as shown in Figure 1.7.

POWER SPECIFICATION OF OPHTHALMIC LENSES

Lenses for camera or other optical instruments are always described in terms of focal length and is given by the equation:

$$F = \frac{1}{FL}$$

Where, F is focal power of the lens
FL is the focal length of the lens in meters.

Ophthalmic lenses, on the hand are described in terms of refracting power. Refracting power is defined as the change in vergence that occurs when light rays passes through a lens. The power of lens describes the extent of change in vergence that happens when the incident wave of light pass through them. Several methods of specifying power of ophthalmic lenses have been used. Some of the common methods are shown in the Flowchart 1.2.

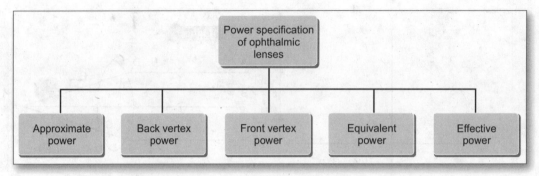

FLOWCHART 1.2: Power specifications of ophthalmic lenses

Approximate Power

The approximate power of the lens is given by the algebraical summation of front surface power of the lens and the back surface power of the lens (Fig. 1.8). The approximate power of the lens is given by the simple equation:

$$Fa = F_1 + F_2$$

Where F_1 is the front surface power and F_2 is the back surface power as given by the curves of the respective surfaces, measured by lens measure watch. Lens measure watch gives the correct surface power only if it has been calibrated to the respective material index. Lens thickness is not considered in this method. That is why the method gives correct power only when the lens thickness is zero, hence it is called approximate power of lens.

Back Vertex Power

Back vertex power (*BVP*) is given by the reciprocal of the posterior vertex focal length multiplied by the refractive index of the lens. The following equation defines the *BVP* of the lens:

$$BVP = \frac{F_1}{1 - \frac{t_c}{n_{lens}}(F_1)} + F_2$$

Where
- F_1 = Front surface power
- F_2 = Back surface power
- t_c = Geometrical center thickness
- n_{lens} = Refractive index of lens material.

In simple terms *BVP* can be defined as the ability of a lens to focus parallel rays with reference to its back pole. Figure 1.9 shows light rays from a distance object is focused by a convex lens at its secondary principal focal point B. The distance from the back vertex pole A to the focal point B, is the back

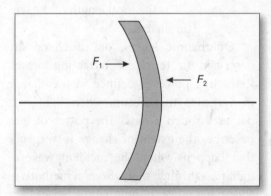

FIGURE 1.8: Front and back surface power as shown by their curves and measured by lens measure watch

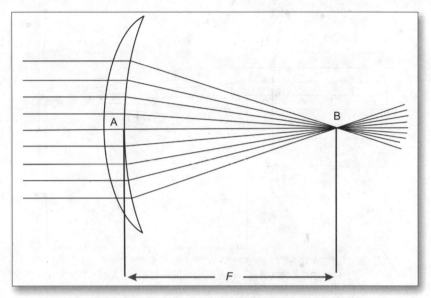

FIGURE 1.9: Back vertex focal length of a plus lens

vertex focal length, given by *F*. When an ophthalmic lens is ordered from a laboratory, it is denoted in terms of its *BVP*. The back vertex focal point for each lens falls at the same distance from the eye and coincides with the patient's far point, correcting the refractive error. The instrument used for measuring the back vertex power of a spectacle lens is the focimeter or lensometer. The reading is taken when a lens is placed on the lensometer with its back vertex in contact with the lens rest.

Front Vertex Power

The distance between the front vertex of the lens A to its first principal focus B is called the front vertex focal length of the lens and the reciprocal of the front vertex focal length of the lens is called front vertex power (*FVP*) of lens (Fig. 1.10). The following equation defines the *FVP* of the lens:

$$FVP = \frac{F_2}{1 - \frac{t_c}{n_{lens}}(F_2)} + F_1$$

Where

- F_1 = Front surface power
- F_2 = Back surface power
- t_c = Geometrical center thickness
- n_{lens} = Refractive index of lens material.

Neutralizing measures the FVP of the lens. Two lenses are said to be neutralized, when placed in contact with each other, their total power is zero. If the lens is placed on the lensometer with its front vertex in contact with the lens rest, the recorded lens power will be *FVP*. *FVP* is measured for segmented bifocal lenses when fused on the convex surface of the lens.

Equivalent Power

Many optical devices are constructed with a series of lenses separated by air or arranged

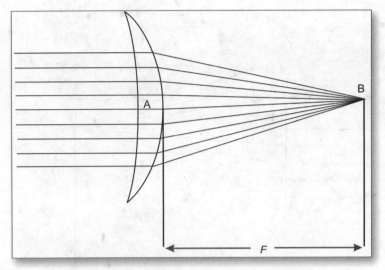

FIGURE 1.10: Front vertex focal length of a plus lens

with a series of curve surfaces separated by medium having different refractive indices. In most of this complex system, the center of curvature of all the surfaces fall on a common optical axis. The entire system so devised is imagined to have one single focal point like a thin lens that would produce an image of distant object of the same size and at the same position as produced by the system. The focal length produced by the system is called equivalent focal length and the reciprocal of focal length in meters is defined as the equivalent power of the lens system.

Effective Power

The effective power of the lens may be defined as the ability of the lens to focus parallel rays of light at a given plane. Plus lens is more effective and brings about more changes in vergence as they move farther away from the eyes (Fig. 1.11) and minus lens becomes less effective as they move farther away from the eyes. Two similar types of lenses having similar *BVP* may have different effective power based upon the vertex distance. It means the effective power of the lens varies with the position of the spectacle frame front on the wearer's face. The lens affectivity formula calculates the effective power of the lens when it is placed at a new distance. The equation is:

$$F' = \frac{F}{1} - dF$$

Where
- F' = Effective power of the lens at its new distance
- F = Effective power of the lens at its initial distance
- d = Change in vertex distance in meters (d is positive if the vertex distance increases and d is negative if vertex distance decreases)

Example: What is the new effective power of a +10.00 D lens if it is moved in by 5 mm?

$$F' = \frac{F}{1} - dF$$

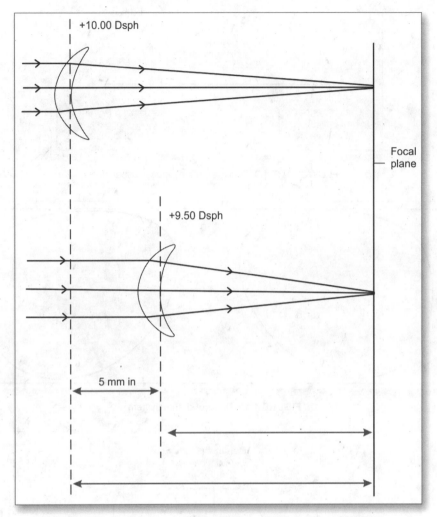

FIGURE 1.11: Change in vertex distance alters effective power of the lens

= +10.00 / 1 − (+ 0.005)(+10.00)
= +9.50 Dsph

SYSTEMS OF OPTICAL DISPENSING

Systems of optical dispensing provide measuring procedures that establish a system of reference points to facilitate accurate lens placement into the frame. There are two systems that are very popular as shown in Flowchart 1.3.

Datum System of Optical Dispensing

Datum system is the British standard for spectacle frame measurements. It provides a system of reference points for frames and lenses to facilitate accurate placement of optical center and bifocal segment height. Two horizontal lines tangent to the top and bottom edges of the lenses are drawn that runs parallel to each other (Fig. 1.12). With reference to those two lines various

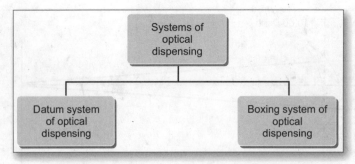

FLOWCHART 1.3: Two systems of optical dispensing

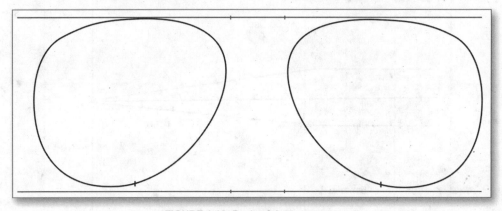

FIGURE 1.12: Basis of datum system

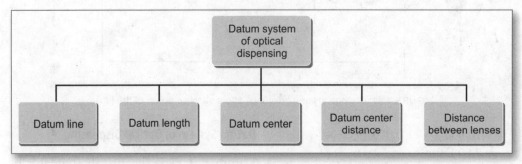

FLOWCHART 1.4: Lens and frame measuring references under datum system

lens and frame measuring references can be explained as shown in Flowchart 1.4.

Datum Line

Datum line is the line that lies midway between the horizontal tangents to lens shape at its top and the bottom edges (Fig.1.13). Datum line of the spectacle frame is continuous with the datum line of each lens.

Datum Length

Datum length is the horizontal measure of the lens shape on its datum line.

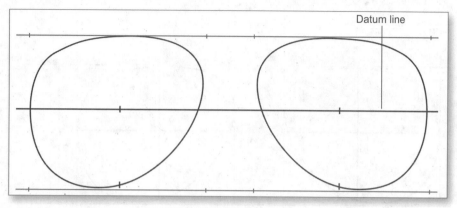

FIGURE 1.13: Datum line

Datum Center

The midpoint lying on datum line denotes the datum center (Fig. 1.14).

Datum Center Distance

Datum center distance is distance between the datum centers of right and left lenses when the lenses are fitted into the frame.

Distance between Lenses

It is the measure of horizontal distance between the nasal edges of the spectacle lenses along the datum line.

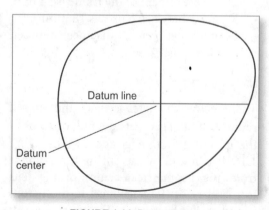

FIGURE 1.14: Datum center

Boxing System of Optical Dispensing

Boxing system is the American standard for spectacle frame measurements. Two vertical lines that are tangent to either side of the lens and run parallel to each other are added, forming a box around the lens as shown in Figure 1.15. With reference to the box so formed important lens and frame measurements as shown in Flowchart 1.5 can be explained.

Geometrical Center

Geometrical center lies at the halfway between the two vertical lines of the box on the datum line. Geometrical center corresponds to the datum center of the British standard. Geometrical center distance (GCD) refers to the distance between the geometric centers of the right and left lens boxes. It can be calculated simply by adding eyewire size to distance between lenses (DBL). It is presumed to be the frame pupillary distance (PD) on the assumption that pupils would correspond to this point. If a frame is marked 52 □ 18, the GCD of the eyewire would be 70 mm.

Size

The size of the lens is given by the length and depth of the box containing the lens.

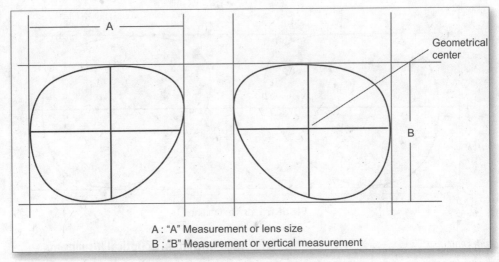

A : "A" Measurement or lens size
B : "B" Measurement or vertical measurement

FIGURE 1.15: Boxing system of measurement

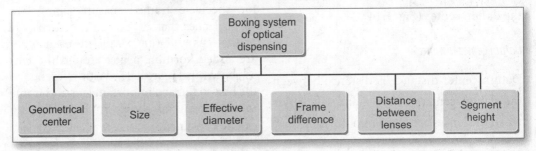

FLOWCHART 1.5: Lens and frame measuring references under boxing system

This denotes the eye size when talked about spectacle frame and lens size when talked about the lens. Horizontal measure of the box is denoted by "A" measurement under boxing system and vertical measurement is denoted by "B" measurement of the box enclosing the lens. "C" measurement refers to the width of the lens itself along the datum line. While measuring the lens size the measurement begins at the apex of the bevel on one side of the lens to the apex of bevel on the opposite side of the lens. While measuring the eye size the measurement begins at the base of the groove on one side of the eyewire to base of the eyewire on the opposite side of the eyewire. Most frames are marked for

their sizes inside of the temple as 54 ☐ 18. The meaning of such notation under boxing system of measurement is:
- "A" Measurement of the frame is 54 mm.
- Distance between lenses is 18 mm.
- Geometrical center distance between two lenses is 72 mm.

Effective Diameter

The effective diameter is twice the longest radius from the geometric center of a lens to the apex of the lens edge as shown in Figure 1.16. It is found by measuring the distance from the geometrical center of the lens to the apex of the lens bevel farthest from it and multiply it by 2. The measurement

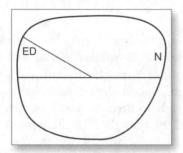

FIGURE 1.16: Effective diameters

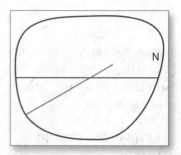

FIGURE 1.17: Effective diameters are measured from optical center to the farthest end of the rim

helps to determine the smallest lens blank from which the lens can be cut. This definition is based on the assumption that the lens optical center will coincide with the geometric center of the frame shape. However, if the lens is decentered towards the nasal direction to match the interpupillary distance of the patient, the longest radius would be measured from the point of optical center to the farthest end of the rim as shown in the Figure 1.17.

Frame Difference

The difference between the horizontal and vertical measurement, measured in millimeter, is known as frame difference. If the frame difference is 0, it implies that the frame eyewire shape is round. If "A" measurement is larger than the "B" measurement, it implies that the frame difference is larger and the shape of the eyewire is rectangular.

Distance between Lenses

DBL is the measure of distance between the nasal vertical tangents to the lenses at the peak of the bevel. It is measured on the frame as the distance from the inside nasal eyewire groove across the bridge area at the narrowest point (Fig. 1.18). This is usually synonymous with the bridge size if the manufacturer follows boxing system of measurement. If a frame is marked with/18\, it implies that the bridge width of the frame is 18 mm.

Segment Height

Datum line or the lower line of the box enclosing the lens shape is mostly used to specify multifocal segment height. The reference is most commonly given as either distance below or above the datum line, or, distance from the lower line of the box

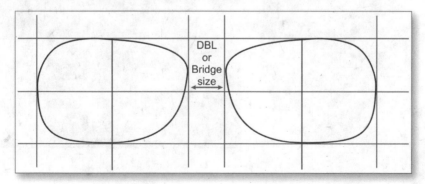

FIGURE 1.18: DBL or bridge size

enclosing the lens shape. For example, in a frame with "A" measurement 51 mm, "B" measurement 47 mm and the segment top is placed 4 mm below datum line, the segment height would be 19.5 mm from the lower line enclosing the lens.

APPLIED ANTHROPOMETRY AND MORPHOLOGY

The spectacle frames are fitted to match both anthropometric and cosmetic demands. The plane of the spectacle frame ideally makes a parallel relation with eyes so that it neither touches eyebrows nor cheeks. Eyes, nose, eyebrows, cheeks, eyelashes, ears and temporal head—all supported by skull are leading organs that plays important roles in the complicated interaction of the spectacle frame and human face. Familiarity with those organs helps frame measurement, frame selection and frame fitting on the face.

Eyes

The round shape eyeball of approximate diameter of 25 mm is placed within the bony socket of the human skull and is visible through almond shaped palpebral aperture. The overall horizontal width of aperture is around 30 mm. Vertical dimension varies from 10 to 12 mm. Palpebral aperture is slightly inclined to the horizontal meridian. The two eyeballs are placed at the same level in most cases. In cases where they are not at the same level, difference in level rarely exceeds 2 mm. There are certain ocular structures like pupil center, limbus, lower eyelid and canthus that are invariably used as reference for various dispensing measurements.

Nose

The relation between frame and the nose crest determines whether the spectacle frame fits comfortably or not. Figures 1.19 and 1.20 show the root, crest, flanks and overall

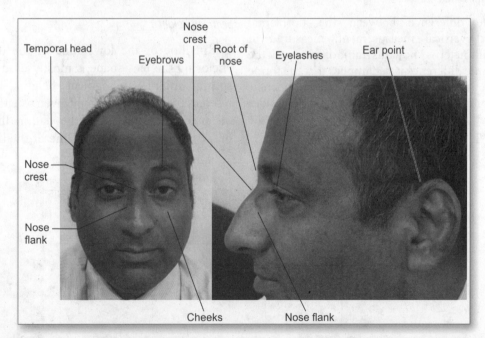

FIGURE 1.19: Facial structures that determine the interaction between spectacle frame and human face

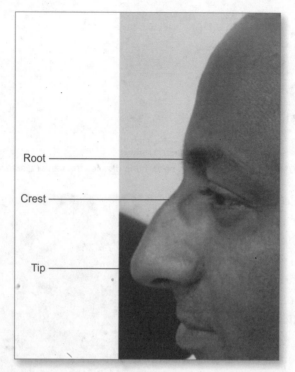

FIGURE 1.20: Crest and root are important parts of nose for spectacle fitting

shape of the nose. They are all important considerations for the comfortable frame fit.

Figure 1.21 shows that the root of the nose is situated at the junction of the nasal and frontal bone and is followed by crest.

The bridge of the nose is the elevation formed by the nasal bones and is the area where the bridge of the spectacle frame rests on the nose crest (Fig. 1.22). The relative levels of the eyes and the bridge of the nose

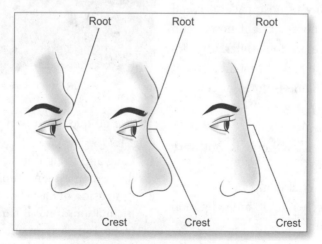

FIGURE 1.21: Different shapes of nose

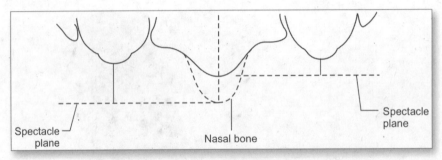

Spectacle plane

Nasal bone

Spectacle plane

FIGURE 1.22: Protrusion of nasal bone dictates the vertex distance

is critical while selecting and fitting the spectacle frame. The protrusion of the nose is measured from a line passing through the apex of the cornea which determines the vertex distance of the spectacle frame front.

The inclination of nasal flanks, both in horizontal and vertical plane is important while fitting the spectacle frame. In the horizontal plane around the level of lower eyelids, splay angle of the nose pads is measured. These features are unique to an individual patient and are important to fit the spectacle frame properly.

There are different types of nose shapes. Each carries certain unique features that influence the fitting of nose pads of metal frames. Concave nose, straight nose, snub nose and flat nose are four different types that affect the nose pads fitting adjustment differently. The unique features of concave nose are (Fig. 1.23):

1. Nose crest is depressed.
2. Protrusion of nasal bone is not very significant.
3. Inclination of nasal flanks in horizontal plane is relatively more than inclination in vertical plane.
4. The tip of the nose is protruded.

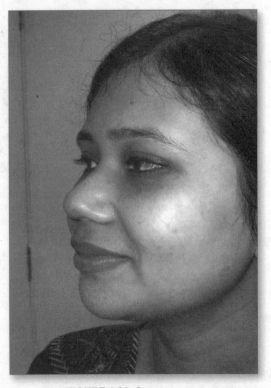

FIGURE 1.23: Concave nose

The unique features of straight nose are (Fig. 1.24):

1. Long and straight nose with no curve or depression is seen at nose crest.
2. Protrusion of nasal bone is significant.
3. Inclination of nasal flanks in horizontal plane is less than inclination of nasal flanks in vertical plane.

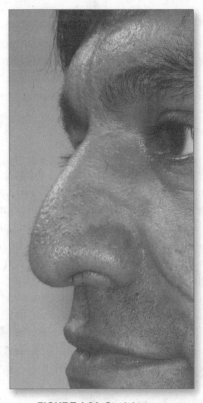

FIGURE 1.24: Straight nose

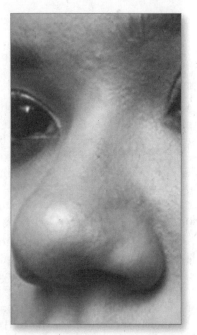

FIGURE 1.25: Snub nose

3. Inclination of nasal flanks in horizontal plane is very large with almost no

4. The tip of the nose is pointed and narrow

The unique features of snub nose are (Fig. 1.25):

1. Small nose relatively depressed nose crest.
2. Protrusion of nasal bone is relatively less.
3. Inclination of nasal flanks in horizontal plane is more than inclination of nasal flanks in vertical plane.
4. The tip of the nose is round and it tends to turn up.

The unique features of flat nose are (Fig. 1.26):

1. Small and flat nose crest.
2. Protrusion of nasal bone is flat with no protrusion.

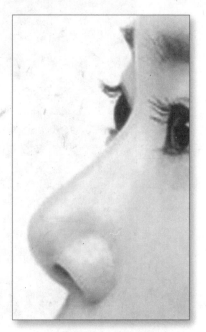

FIGURE 1.26: Flat nose

inclination of nasal flanks in vertical plane.

4. The tip of the nose is flared and wide.

Eyebrows

The shape and position of eyebrows determines the shape of the eyewear that will suit a wearer. An ideal choice is based on the fact that the upper rim of the front of the frame should be either below or in line with the position of the eyebrows.

Cheeks

The position of the cheeks relative to the bridge of the nose determines the inclination of the front of the frame through the angle of sides. A more pronounced cheek is critical to note while adjusting the frame-front for vertical angle. Vertical angle of the frame is adjusted so as to ensure that the lower eyewire does not make any contact with the cheeks.

Eyelashes

The length of the eyelashes of the upper lid determines the minimum vertex distance of the spectacle lens. Ideally eyelashes should never make contact with back surface of the lens.

Ears

The position of the ears beyond the plane of the nose bridge determines the overall length of the sides of the frame. Their position in the vertical plane also determines the angle of the sides. The ear point lies at the bearing surface of the temple bend. Most ears are set close enough to the head to provide a definite crotch into which the sides can be fitted. They are of great importance to fit the spectacle frame for length to bend, angle of the drop and pantoscopic tilt. Figure 1.27 shows the different shapes of the ear that

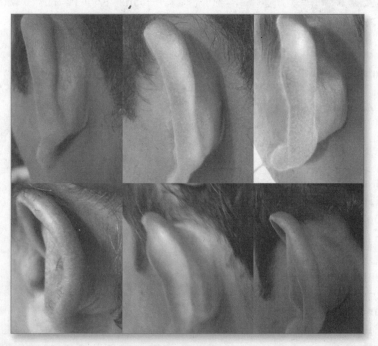

FIGURE 1.27: Different shapes of ears that affects angle of the drop of the temple bend

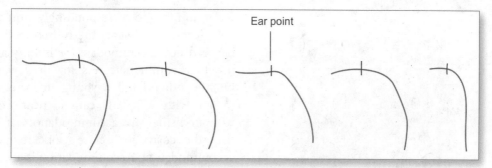

FIGURE 1.28: Different ways the angle of the drop of temple bend can be made

affects the angle of the drop of the temple bend as shown by Figure 1.28.

Temporal Head

The distance between right and left temporal head of the wearer's head, measured at a level approximately 25–30 mm behind the nose crest plane around the ears (Fig. 1.29) provides facial width which determines the required temple width of the spectacle frame. The measured temple width of the frame has to conform with facial width of the wearer so that the temples when running through the sides of the face makes parallel relation with the temporal bones and makes contact only on top of the ears.

It is important to understand that a number of variations can be seen as far as the shape of human skull is concerned. However, there is one unique aspect that is being observed commonly in most people, i.e. the anterior part of the head is wedge-shaped. The plane of the face normally represents the narrowest that gradually becomes widest around the ear point and is followed by another wedge-shaped part of the skull that points away from the face as shown in Figure 1.30.

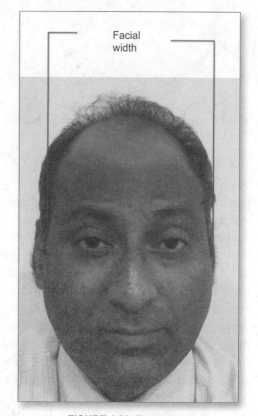

FIGURE 1.29: Facial width

PSYCHOLOGY OF DISPENSING

More than 90% of information we receive is through vision. Our vision system is driven by the evolution of visual behavior that enables us to be capable of perceiving

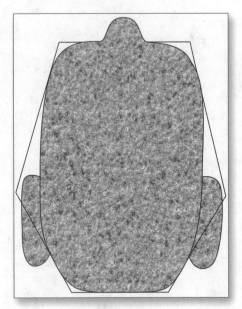

FIGURE 1.30: Wedge-shaped head as seen from the top

and then reacting to the environment continuously. Over a period of time a person develops a visual behavior pattern. When the lenses are worn, lot of changes happen in the visual system and the first-time wearer needs to make some changes in his developed visual behavior. The first-time wearer may also feel some unusual sensation. He may feel that the new lenses are "too strong", or he may notice some changes in depth of perception. Moreover, he may find himself more conscious about the new correction, finding it difficult to coordinate with head and eye movement specially with his new presbyopic correction. A young adult with the small amount of correction may also feel "pulling sensation" which may be associated with the need to establish a new relationship between accommodation and convergence mechanism of the visual system. A young uncorrected hyperope with +2.50 D accommodates by that amount to

see at infinity and correspondingly more for near work. If he wears the full correction, he need not accommodate for infinity and has to accommodate less for near work. On the other hand a young uncorrected myope with − 2.50 D can do near work without using any accommodation. If he uses the correction, close work requires accommodation. Accommodation is always associated with convergence. Thus, excess convergence is also relaxed when a hyperope uses correction, whereas correction in myopia stimulates convergence. The straight forward meaning is the person needs to make changes in his visual habits and changes require sustained efforts to overcome the initial difficulties.

When a spectacle lens is worn, a series of changes is noticed in visual performance. Some of these changes are intended and others come along. A notable behavior change is seen in the wearer as plus lens wearer emphasizes more on ground because of expanded space horizon. On the contrary, a minus lens wearer emphasizes more on figure because of constricted space horizon. A plus lens wearer is peripherally more aware, whereas minus lens wearer finds himself good at central detailing. Plus lenses spread light scatter and decrease light intensity and minus lenses decrease light scatter and increase light intensity. This could be a reason, why an optimally corrected hyperope with optimum vision will always find his contrast reduced more than the optimally corrected myope with optimum vision. Some sensitive wearer may feel changes in perception of spatial orientation. While some people are lucky and can see well, for many people adapting to these changes may not come easy. Understanding the elements of change, the stages of change and ways to work through each stage may help the wearer to achieve desired goals. No single solution works for everyone, often you need to resort to trial and error method in order to achieve the desired goals. It is during this period, that many people are discouraged and give up. The key to success is to stay motivated and follow the advice of the optician. One of the most important things that the patient needs to do is to give up complaining during the initial period of adaptation and make a sincere try before jumping onto any conclusion.

Getting used to a new prescription or a new multifocal lens requires a patient to break his visual habits of past and develop a new habit that compliments to the new lens type. It means educating the patient is the key for successful adaptation. The better the patient understands what he needs to do, the better are the chances of success. With a new pair of lenses, things may not appear perfect initially, but eventually it has to be perfect. The process of adaptation is similar to breaking into a new pair of shoes. If your spectacle is first ever, the best way to get used to them is to wear them as often as possible or as directed by your optometrist. Using them in small doses unnecessarily delays the adaptation. Adapting to new lenses is normal. By providing a thorough understanding to all parties and patience, the adaptation process can run much smoother for both the patient and practitioner. As a dispensing optician you need to have a working knowledge of applied psychology. Sharing knowledge helps your patients' understand the condition and maintain the required enthusiasm to adapt to the new lenses.

Moreover, there are barriers to the use of spectacle also. This is obvious when you notice that vision is the most neglected aspect of healthcare. Most people believe that their vision is absolutely perfect until their problem manifests and starts affecting their visual performances. This is because of the adapting ability of the visual system. The visual system does not handicap the process of understanding the environment in which we live. The obvious deficiency in the process of vision slows down gradually until the responses start causing confusion, poor performance and then frustration. If a child performs poor in reading, it is normally taken to be the problem related to his ability. Vision is most often the last thing to blame. Besides, there is a class of people who believe that wearing spectacles creates social barrier, affecting social life and the economic prospects of an individual by restricting the educational and employment opportunities. Girls are particularly vulnerable to social and psychological distress. Even the children had been victimized of negative perception about spectacle. If a child complains of not been able to see the blackboard in the classroom, the grandparents in the family say that he is feigning to wear spectacles. Attitude like this could result in serious problems like psychosocial maladjustments.

Looking at such a typical scenario it may appear difficult and somewhat gloomy; nevertheless, the adequate correction of refractive error in itself is interesting and brings lot of satisfaction. It also eliminates disabilities both in work and play than any other single method technique.

POINTS TO REMEMBER

- Human eye is most sensitive to yellow color.
- Light with longest wavelength detected by our eyes is perceived as red color.
- Pluslenses are the combination of prisms base to base while minus-lenses are the combination of prisms apex to apex.
- When light strikes the lens surface, some of the light is lost because of absorption, some of the light is reflected back to the same medium and most proportion of the light is transmitted.
- The two principal meridians of ophthalmic lenses are known as axis meridian and power meridian. Axis meridian has the minimum lens power and power meridian has the maximum lens power.
- Reciprocal of focal length of the lens in meter is known as the lens power.
- Lens laboratory denotes the power of ophthalmic lenses in terms of BVP of the lens.
- A line drawn halfway between the top edge of the lens and the bottom edge of the lens and is parallel to them is known as datum line.
- Center point on the datum line and halfway between the two vertical lines is known as geometrical center.
- The concept of boxing system is based upon the idea of drawing an imaginary box around a lens shape with the box's side's tangent to the outer most edges of the lens shape. The system uses the sides of the boxes as reference points for drawing various standards for measurements.
- "A" measurement in boxing system refers to the horizontal measure of the lens.
- "B" measurement in boxing system refers to the vertical measure of the lens.
- Frame difference is the difference between the horizontal and the vertical measurements, measured in millimeter.
- The larger the frame difference the shape of the lens would be narrow rectangular.
- When the frame difference is 0, the shape of the lens would be round.
- The effective diameter of a lens is twice the longest radius from the geometric center of the lens to the apex of the lens bevel farthest from it.
- The measurement of effective diameter helps to determine the smallest lens blank from which the lens can be cut.
- The geometrical center distance is same as the eye size + bridge size.
- The protrusion of the nose is measured from a line passing through the apex of the cornea which determines the vertex distance of the spectacle frame front.
- The position of the ears beyond the plane of the nose bridge determines the overall length of the sides of the frame.

CHAPTER 2

FRAME TYPES AND FRAME MATERIALS

Spectacle frames are today more than just an eyewear to hold the lens in position. They differ not only by style but also by materials. The objective of this chapter is to acquaint the reader with different frame styles or types that are available and applications of different materials used to manufacture the frames. Understanding frame styles need power of authenticity, passion of detailing and a cult of creativity.

Spectacle frames have a long history that has evolved from crude and heavy contrivances to the comfortable devices of modern times. Modern frames are made of diversified materials in diversified designs and are made using very sophisticated technology.

The process starts with creative work of the design studio and finishes with turning the design drafts into real spectacle frame. This is not an easy task and is very often a challenging one. The entire manufacturing process may require well over 150 operations including dozens of inspection process.

FRAME TYPES

Spectacle frames are made of metal, plastic or any other material; that features a front and two temples that reach behind the ears. Several types of spectacle frames are available. Basically they differ in the way they are being designed to look. Some of the most common frame types are shown in the Flowchart 2.1.

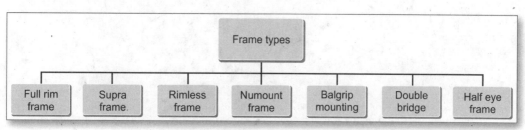

FLOWCHART 2.1: Different types of frames

Full Rim Frame

Full rim frames are the most common frames type that are made with either plastic material or metal or combination of both or any other material in various shapes and sizes. The lenses are surrounded by the rim or eyewire from all around (Fig. 2.1). Full rim frames are made in variety of shapes. Some of the common shapes are aviator, square, rectangle, oval, panto and many unique shapes specially designed for females.

Supra Frame

Supra frames are most commonly called half rim frames in which the lenses are secured using nylon monofilament to the semi-rimless chassis. The cord is attached to the top half rim or eyewire and a groove is cut into the lens edge that serves as a channel into which the nylon monofilament fits (Fig. 2.2). Supra frames differ with rimway frames, as the rimway frames have two holes per lens and a metal reinforcing wire that follows the upper posterior surface of the lens.

Rimless Frame

The rimless assembly consists of a bridge, a pair of temples and two end pieces, i.e. three parts in total (Fig. 2.3). It is for this reason they are also known as "three piece" frames. Mostly they are made of metal material. The temples and the bridge are attached directly to the lens either with screw and hex nuts or prongs, barbs and specialized bushes or fixing pins or others. The new technology mounts the lenses using new compression tools. The process of lens mounting is simple and the total assembly is less stressful than screws and nuts. Bushing cushions lens'

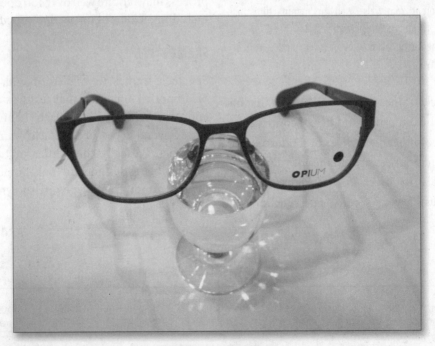

FIGURE 2.1: Full rim frame

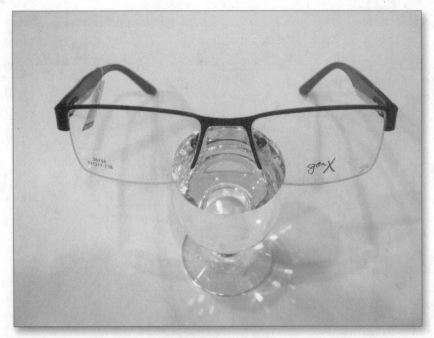

FIGURE 2.2: Supra frame

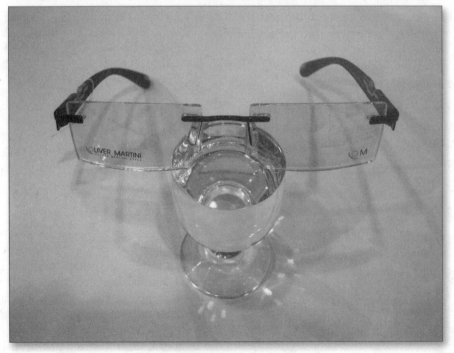

FIGURE 2.3: Rimless frame

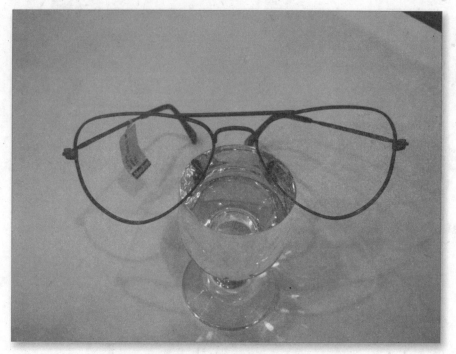

FIGURE 2.4: Double bridge frame

lateral movement and hence minimizes the chances of lens cracking around the drilled holes.

Double Bridge Frame

Some frames are designed with a reinforcing bar that crosses the top of the eyewire or the lenses (Fig. 2.4). This is very popular in aviator shape. It acts as an additional support for the frame and also provides a new style.

Balgrip Mounting Frame

Balgrip mounting holds the lens in place with the help of clip attached to the rim made of tensile metal that fits into nasal and temporal slot on each side of lens as shown in Figure 2.5. The lenses can be removed easily by pulling the clip out from the lens slot. Even the wearer can remove the lens and fit them again.

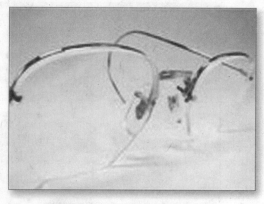

FIGURE 2.5: Balgrip mounting frame

Numount Frame

Numount frames are usually made in metal material. It consists of upper half rim, bridge and two temples. The lenses are attached only at their nasal area. Temples are attached to the top metal eyewire that extends along the temporal skull to reach behind the ears (Fig. 2.6).

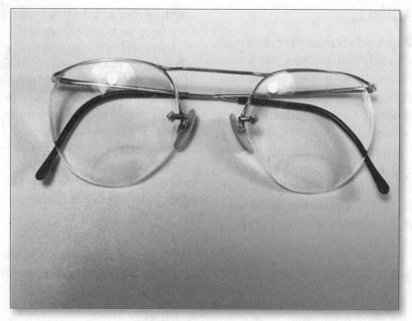

FIGURE 2.6: Numount frame

Half Eye Frame

Half eye frames, also known as reading frames are meant for people who need only near correction. They are typically worn slightly down on the nose so that the line of sight does not pass through the lens while looking at any distant object (Fig. 2.7).

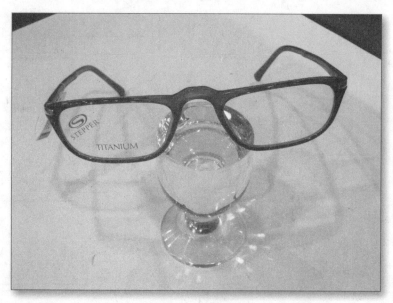

FIGURE 2.7: Half eye frame

FRAME MATERIALS

When the spectacle frames were developed, they were mostly made of precious materials like tortoise shell, gold or buffalo horn. It is only after the advances in manufacturing technology of mass-production, wide varieties of materials were tried with an objective to improve the machinability of the material, reduce the cost of production, and improve craftsmanship. Mostly plastic and metal family of materials as shown in Flowchart 2.2 are used to manufacture the spectacle frames.

Plastic Frames

Plastic material is the most commonly used material for mass production of spectacle frames. Plastics are synthetic polymers and may be grouped into two broad categories: Theromoplastic and thermosetting.

Thermoplastic materials are linear polymers, they flow on heating. Thermosetting materials are crosslinked polymers, they do not flow on heating. Once molded and set in a shape, they cannot be reshaped or remolded. Most materials used for plastic frames manufacturing are of thermoplastic variety. Among all the plastic materials used for spectacle frame manufacturing, the following are most common:

Celluloid Nitrate

Celluloid nitrate is a thermoplastic material. Spectacle frames are made from flat sheets of celluloid material.

Advantages

• The material polishes well.

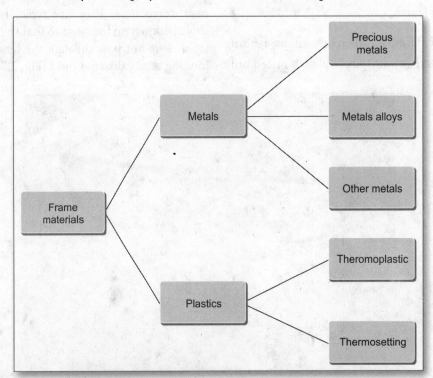

FLOWCHART 2.2: Types of materials used for spectacle frames

- The strong machinability of the material makes it easy to work with.

Disadvantages

- The color of the material fades quickly.
- The material dries up soon and becomes brittle.
- The material is highly inflammable.
- It softens faster with heat and excessive heating causes blistering and rolling of rims.

Recommended system for lens insertion

- Use of an air heater or a salt pan is recommended for lens insertion.
- Avoid overheating.
- The temperature of your warmer should be controlled and should not exceed 70°C.

Celluloid Acetate

Celluloid acetate is a thermoplastic material. Spectacle frames are made from flat sheets of celluloid material.

Advantages

- The material polishes well.
- The material is easy to work with.
- Colors can be produced in multiple layers. Enormous range of colors is possible. Carving reveals different colors.

Disadvantages

- The material deteriorates over time and forms a layer of white surface.
- It cracks and becomes brittle with time.
- The material softens with heat and shrinks slightly.
- Excess heating will cause blistering and rolling of rim.

Recommended system for lens insertion

- Use of an air heater or a salt pan is recommended for lens insertion.

- Avoid overheating.
- The temperature of your warmer should be controlled and should not exceed 70°C.
- Older frames material looses flexibility and therefore they should be heated thoroughly, but carefully.
- It is recommended to heat only the part of the frame requiring adjustment and submerging only the heated portion into water.

Celluloid Propionate

Celluloid propionate is a thermoplastic material. Spectacle frames are made by forced injection molding process.

Advantages

- Cost of production is cheaper as fewer steps are required and the waste is less.
- Wide colors are possible with dip coating process.
- The material is very durable for longer period of use.
- The material is very heat sensitive.
- The material is not well-suited for stretching or shrinking.

Disadvantages

Material uses more plasticizers which make it more sensitive to heat.

Recommended system for lens insertion

- It is recommended to use an air heater as opposed to a salt pan to allow more controlled heat application.
- The maximum working temperature for this material should not exceed 40°C.
- Lenses should be edged to very close tolerance since this material is not well-suited to stretching or shrinking.

Nylon

Nylon is a thermoplastic material. Spectacle frames are made by forced injection molding process.

Advantages

- The material is easy to mold to frame shapes.
- Nylon is very ideal for eyewear. It provides minimal weight with high strength.
- It provides stability of shapes even in hot environment.
- Nylon material can be used to make thinner eye wire frames.
- They also provide better anatomical fit at the nose.
- It is possible to make transparent and glossy surface finish.
- Frame coloring is possible by dip coating procedure. Final touch of coloring may be given by printing, which can also make sophisticated patterns.

Disadvantages

Nylon material dries out due to low humidity. It is, therefore, recommended that the wearer soak the frame in water overnight on a periodic basis. This will prolong frame life and deter breakage.

Recommended system for lens insertion

- The material softens very fast on heating.
- It is recommended to use an air heater as opposed to a salt pan to allow more controlled heat application.
- Apply high heat to adjust the frame and submerge only the newly heated portion into very cold water.

Carbon Fiber

Carbon fiber frames are another type of material used to manufacture frames by injection-molded technology. The material has a better balance between light weight, strength and durability. The most common application of this material is in making combination frame with a carbon front and a metal temple or metal front and carbon temples. These frames deliver the look of an ultra thin plastic frame while exhibiting many of the characteristics of a metal frame.

Advantages

- Carbon fiber frames exhibit good shape retention, light weight and strength.
- Since carbon is black, coloring of these frames is achieved through enameling process.

Disadvantages

Changes in the carbon portion are not readily achieved. Hence pantoscopic and retroscopic adjustments should be provided from the metal portion of the end piece rather than the carbon material itself.

Recommended system for lens insertion

- Lenses for carbon material front should be sized exactly and should be "cold snap" inserted.
- Some carbon frame fronts are also designed to have screws like metal frames for lens insertion.

Optyl

Optyl is an epoxy resin. The material was specially developed to manufacture spectacle frames. Frames are made from this material by a process of casting and then curing. After the finishing operations, frames are dyed in liquid colors. Polishing is done by immersing in a bath of polyurethane.

Advantages

- The material is very light in weight.
- The material allows to maintain rigidity and stability in its "set or adjusted" state.

Disadvantages

The material is very brittle.

Recommended system for lens insertion:

- It needs lot of heat and then suddenly goes very soft.
- It can absorb heat as much as 200°C and then come back to its original shape.
- Use bead pan or air blower to apply heat.
- After inserting the lens, do not put into the water. Allow cooling outside the water, it will come to its original shape.
- Only heat the portion that needs to be adjusted.

Metal Frames

Metal frames are usually made of metal alloys specially developed to suit the skin. In fact most base metals oxidize and corrode easily and react variably. In order to avoid this problem, alloy of two or more metals is made in which the major component is one type of metal. The aim of making alloy is generally to make the material less brittle, hard and resistant to corrosion or have a more desirable color and luster. Metal by its nature are malleable that allows working with its shape through the pressure and torque applied gently using plier. A metal spectacle frame uses various combinations of metal materials to create the most functional design. One metal may be chosen

for an end piece because of its rigidity, while on the same frame a different flexible metal is chosen for the temple, and yet another metal may be chosen as a final finish because of its hardness or luster. In general, following metal materials are commonly used for spectacle frames:

A. Precious metals
   1. Gold
   2. Silver
   3. White gold.
B. Metal alloys
   1. Rolled gold
   2. Nickel alloys
   3. Monel alloys.
C. Other metals
   1. Titanium
   2. Aluminium
   3. Stainless steel.

Precious Metals

Gold and silver are most common precious metals used for exclusive metal eyewear. Apart from its value and noble appearance gold has lot of other merits. Gold is highly resistance to tarnishing and corrosion and can be shaped to any style and thickness with ease. The only disadvantage is that the gold in its purest form is very soft and has to be alloyed with other metals to add needed strength and hardness. Gold alloyed with other metals is known as carat gold and is designated as so many carats according to the proportion of gold in the alloy. 24 ct is termed as pure gold, and the purity goes down to 18 ct, 12 ct and 9 ct. The higher qualities are more resistant to corrosion and are more valuable. The proportion of other metal in the alloy determines the effective color appearance of the gold frames. A pink effect is obtained by increasing the proportion of copper. White gold is obtained by replacing silver with nickel and copper with zinc. A white finish can also be obtained by electroplating gold material with another precious metal rhodium. Other precious metals used are palladium and rhodium which are silvery finish, hard and very expensive.

Metal Alloys

Rolled gold—Rolled gold is designed to provide most of the advantage of gold at cheaper cost. A thin plate or plates of gold is welded to a block of base metal. The adjoining surface is carefully milled to ensure even contact. After the materials have been bonded together the block is subjected to cold-rolling process in order to reduce the gold layer to desired thinness The material is then drawn or formed into wire, strip or tubing having an even covering of carat gold. Bronze and nickel silver are mostly preferred alloys. The gold content depends upon two things— the purity of gold cladding and the proportion of gold covering to base metal. The usual way of expressing the gold quality is "1/10th 10 ct" which implies that the skin is made of 10 ct gold and accounts for 1/10th of the total weight of the whole material. The end product is eventually gold plated to improve the appearance of final product.

Nickel silver—The nickel silver contains as little as 12–25% nickel and mostly copper. The proportion of silver may be very negligible or sometimes no silver. Mechanically this is an excellent metal alloy for spectacle frames and is fairly resistant to corrosion. If not plated or coated it rapidly turns green in contact with bodily fluids. It can be easily worked to any shape and soldered. It is,

therefore, the most common material for the spectacle frames. Nickel silver alloy is also used very commonly for making joints and side's reinforcement of plastic frames.

Monel alloy—This is similar to nickel silver, but contains 68% of nickel. The higher nickel content reduces the rate of corrosion.

Other Metals

Titanium—Titanium is probably closest to the most ideal metal material for the spectacle frames because of its following properties:

1. Mechanically very strong.
2. Corrosion resistant and is not affected by perspiration.
3. Light weight and hypoallergenic in its purest form.

Currently they are very expensive for spectacle frames which do not seem to be associated with the manufacturing costs. It is relatively difficult to plate with more attractive metals such as gold. Sometimes they are colored by a process called "ion plating" which is very much similar to vacuum coating of lenses.

It should be noted titanium frames are seldom made completely with pure titanium material. Screws, nose pads and side tips are frequently excluded. There are other descriptors, such as, β-titanium in which only about 75–80% is titanium, the rest being either aluminium, chromium, iron, molybdenum, niobium, zirconium, etc.

Aluminium—Aluminium is very light and soft and in its pure form it is hypoallergenic and is highly resistant to corrosion. Aluminium parts are always quite thick for a metal frame, due to the softness of the material. Being a good conductor of heat, aluminium is noticeably cold to the touch. It can be beautifully decorated by a process known as anodizing.

Stainless steel—Stainless steel is relatively difficult to work with and is highly resistant to corrosion. It is relatively uncommon material for spectacle frame, although their use is increasing.

METALS USED FOR PLATING METAL FRAMES

Gold, palladium, rhodium, chromium, nickel, silver, copper, etc. are most commonly used for plating the metal frames. Gold is used as an alloy, frequently with silver and copper, platinum group metals like palladium and rhodium are used to provide silvery metal finish. Chromium is also silvery metal. Nickel, silver and copper are very often used as an intermediate layer to improve the adherence and elasticity.

LACQUERING OF FRAMES

The majority of metal frames and some plastic frames are now covered with an organic material either to reduce surface corrosion or for cosmetic reasons. These lacquers can be either applied as a liquid or as a powder which is then heated on metal frames until it liquefies. They are either polymerized before application or during heating process. Common polymers include polyurethanes, polymethylmethacrylate and epoxy resins.

POINTS TO REMEMBER

- Full rim frames are defined by a bridge with two eyewire shapes surrounding the lenses from all around.
- Supra frames hold the lenses in place by means of a nylon cord that fits around the edge of the lenses, giving the frame an appearance of rimless frame.
- Rimway frames have two holes per lens and a metal reinforcing wire that follows the upper posterior surface of the lens.
- Balgrip frames are those that secure the lenses in place with clips attached to a bar of tensile metal that fits into a slot on each side of the lenses.
- Numount frames hold the lenses in place only at their nasal edge.
- Half eye frames are those frames that are meant for people who need a near vision correction only.
- Titanium in its purest form is mechanically very strong, corrosion resistant, light weight and hypoallergic.
- Carbon fiber belongs to plastic material family that is used to manufacture spectacle frames but cannot be obtained in a transparent form.
- Polyurethane is commonly used for lacquer coating of metal frames.
- Stainless steel is so called because of its high corrosion resistance ability.

PARTS OF THE SPECTACLE FRAME

There are different parts that are combined together to make a spectacle frame. Each part serves a specific function and has distinct importance. Knowing the function and application of these parts are very critical for successful dispensing of spectacle. The objective of Chapter 3 is to bring an insight on the application of different parts of the frame.

The spectacle frame has to fit comfortably to the wearer so that it can be used for a longer period of time. In order to ensure ideal fitting, the spectacle frame is adjusted from its various parts. A detail knowledge of the parts as shown in Flowchart 3.1 is very important to understand their functional importance for spectacle dispensing.

FRAME FRONTS

The part of the frame that houses the lens and allows the wearer to see through them is called frame front (Fig. 3.1).

Eyewire

The eyewire or rims are the part of the frame front that surrounds the lens. The eyewire

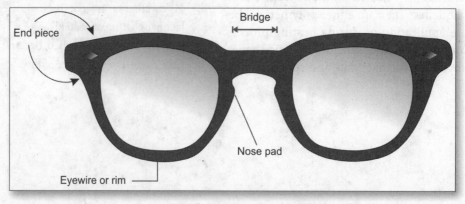

FIGURE 3.1: Frame front

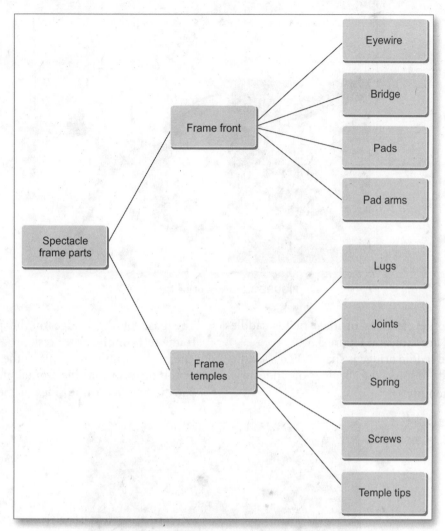

FLOWCHART 3.1: Parts of spectacle frames

thickness depends upon material and design of the frame. The thicker eyewire or rim of plastic frames hides the lens thickness within itself and are designed without any joints, whereas eyewire or rim forming in metal frames is designed with joints where the upper and the lower rims meet at the closing blocks and are joined together with screws.

Bridge

The bridge of the frame connects the right eyewire of the front to the left eyewire of the front. In plastic frames it is shaped to act as the bearing surface on the wearer's nose (Fig. 3.2). The width of the bridge determines the frontal angle in case of plastic frame.

There are two types of bridge that are quite common in plastic frames. They are:
- Saddle bridge
- Keyhole bridge.

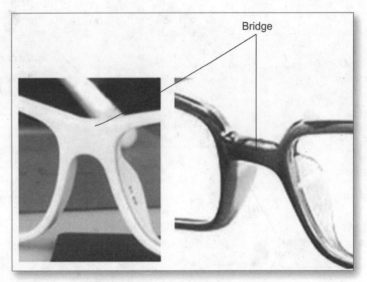

FIGURE 3.2: Bridge of the frame

The key features of ideal fit for saddle bridge are shown in Figure 3.3.
- The saddle bridge is shaped like a saddle and follows the bridge of the nose smoothly.

- The base of the bridge of the plastic frame rests on the nose crest.
- The bridge width conforms to the width of the nose so that the frontal angle of pads is parallel to the sides of the nose

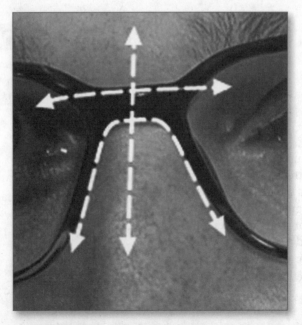

FIGURE 3.3: Ideal fitting of saddle bridge

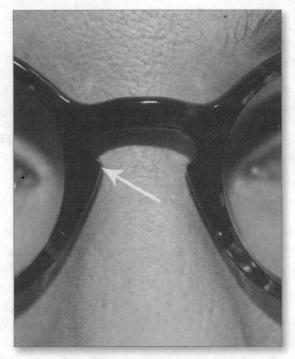

FIGURE 3.4: Keyhole bridge

and the total weight of the spectacle frame is distributed on the wider bearing surface both in horizontal and vertical plane of nasal flank.

Keyhole bridge makes contact only at two points on the sides of the nose as shown in Figure 3.4.

Pads

Pads or nose pads are attached to the pad arms to rest on the nose and provide cushion to bear the entire weight of the metal frame such that the metal rims of the front does not come in contact with skin. They are made of either rigid plastics or silicone material but have a metallic insert for the attachment to pad arms. There are different types of pads as shown in Figure 3.5.

- Rocking pads
- Adjustable strap pads
- Fixed form pads.

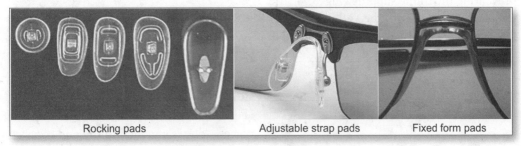

Rocking pads   Adjustable strap pads   Fixed form pads

FIGURE 3.5: Different types of pads

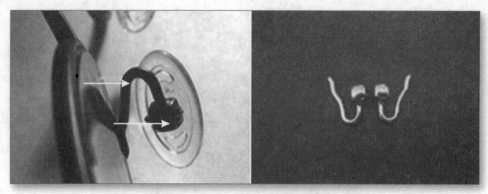

FIGURE 3.6: Pad arms

Fixed form pads do not allow any sort of adjustments possibility, whereas rocking pads allow to make necessary adjustments for splay angle, frontal angle and vertical angle.

Pad Arms

The two small pads are attached to the eyewire with pad arms. These pad arms are located just under the bridge on the nasal side of the eyewire and are attached with point soldering (Fig. 3.6). Pad arms allow modification for vertical angle of nose pads.

TEMPLES

Temples, also known as earpieces, arms or sides are the second most important part of the frames that extend over and/or behind the ears to hold the frame in place, preventing the frame slipping (Fig. 3.7). The temples are joined with the end piece of the front by joints A. The portion of the temple

from A to B in Figure 3.7 is the thickest, portion of the temple that is the nearest attachment to the front is known as butt. The portion on the temple from C to point D where it first bends down to go over the ear at point C is called the bend. The portion BC that lies between the butt and the bend is called the shaft and the portion near the joint is referred to as end piece. While dispensing two different fitting adjustments can be done using temples—temple curve and temple bend.

Lugs

Lugs are also known as end piece. They are extension at each end of the frame front to which the joints or sides or temples are attached (Fig. 3.8). This is the portion from where pantoscopic angle of the frame is modified.

Joints

Joints are the means of attachment for the sides with the front on which they can pivot (Fig. 3.9). All the joints are made of two pieces—one is attached to the end pieces of the front and another is attached to temples.

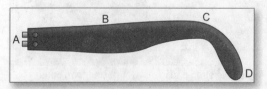

FIGURE 3.7: Temple of spectacle frame

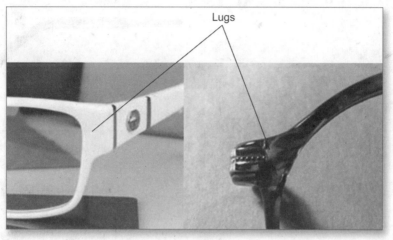

FIGURE 3.8: Lugs

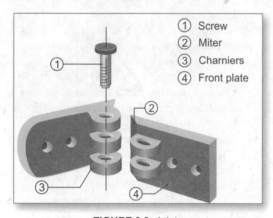

① Screw
② Miter
③ Charniers
④ Front plate

FIGURE 3.9: Joints

Spring Loaded Joints

Spring loaded joints allow outstretching of the temples to predefined extent without damaging the joints and ensuring an elastic stop (Fig. 3.10). Spring loaded joints allows the temples to press against the wearer's temple head so that the frame is secured more tightly and to enable the wearer to use the spectacle frame more comfortably without slipping tendency.

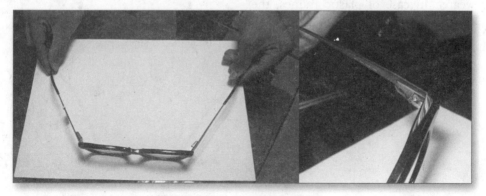

FIGURE 3.10: Spring loaded joints

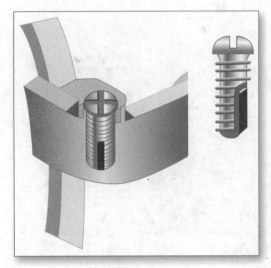

FIGURE 3.11: Screws

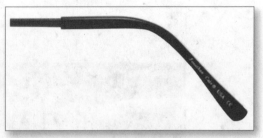

FIGURE 3.12: Tips

Screws

Screws are the smallest part of the frames (Fig. 3.11). Some manufacturer places silicone on the screw thread and when the screw is tightened, the silicone expands between the thread of the closing block and the screws, thus ensuring good friction.

Temple Tips

Temple tips are usually removable plastic sleeves that slip over the ends of metal temples (Fig. 3.12) to provide comfort for the wearer. In case of plastic frames, the temple tip is the part of the temple that goes behind the ears.

POINTS TO REMEMBER

- The saddle bridge is shaped like a saddle and follows the bridge of the nose smoothly.
- Saddle bridge spreads the weight of the frame evenly over the sides and crest of the nose.
- The type of bridge that rests on the sides of the nose, but not on the crest is known as keyhole bridge.
- The type of nose pads fitted in the metal frame that does not allow any sort of adjustments possibility is known as fixed form pads.
- Removable sleeves that slip over the ends of the metal temples are known as temple tips.
- The portion of the temple that is the nearest attachment to the front is known as butt.
- The portion on the temple where it first bends down to go over the ear is called the bend.
- The portion between the butt and the bend is called the shaft.

FRAME SELECTION

Personal products like spectacle frames and sunglasses are now defined as the expression of one's self. But selecting an appropriate frame is not an easy task, because not all frames are equally good for all faces, not all frames matches equally to all prescription and not all frames serves equal function ability. The objective of Chapter 4 is to acquaint the reader with a guideline for careful selection of frames that can make a difference to the way you look and see the world.

The increasing complexities of lifestyle and ever changing aspirational values have changed the way people look at their eyewear or spectacle frame. Today in modern society eyewear is no more a tool to hold the lenses only. They are also the fashion accessories. A frame has to look good and also provide maximum wearing comfort. People like to express themselves by their eyewear. You can blend in or stand out in a crowd; you can have an intellectual look or something very modern and stylish.

A rightly selected frame can actually enhance your features or compensate for not so good facial feature to make you look good. For a dispensing optician frame selection entails much more than just helping a person try on frames. In fact this is the most important function of the dispensing optician. The secret of success in optical dispensing lies in the art of frame selection. People often forget that having eyes examined by an expert professional is just one part of correction. If the spectacle frames are not correctly selected and fitted then even the best refraction will not provide the desired results. It implies that a dispensing optician needs to go beyond the paradigm of techniques and science of dispensing to understand the basic conceptions of shapes, colors and styles. Based upon above concept, it is possible to devise fundamental laws as shown in Flowchart 4.1, which can be used to propose a guideline for appropriate frame selection.

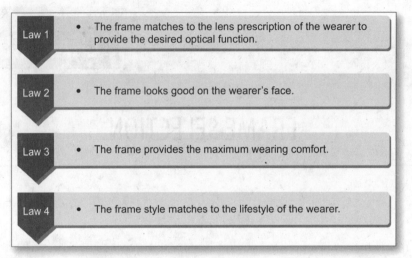

FLOWCHART 4.1: Laws of spectacle frame selection

The frame matches to the lens prescription of the wearer to provide the desired optical function.

This is based on the conception that not all frame styles are equally appropriate for each lens prescription. Frames as the means for carrying the lenses is critically important in dispensing to transfer the clinical findings into reality. The wearer needs to understand that frames vary in their shape, size and style and an inappropriate selection can make things significantly compromised in terms of visual performance through the lenses. The straight forward implication is that the potential for improvement is enormous with an appropriate frame selection.

The frame looks good on the wearer's face.

Looking good is important. The hypothesis is that anything that does not look good is not used. It is, therefore, important that the frame does not make the wearer feel out of date or conspicuous.

The frame provides the maximum wearing comfort.

This is based on the assumption that a frame that fits well also provides the maximum wearing comfort. Disadvantages like frame slipping and tight fit should be minimized. If the spectacle frames are uncomfortable, the wearer will be aware of it that will distract him from other behavioral responses.

The frame style matches to the lifestyle of the wearer.

This is based upon conception that one style does not fit to all occasions or does not serve all purpose. Most people would not like to restrict to one style or look. Understanding lifestyle is the key to cater specific needs which includes occupations, recreations and other concerns like wearer's likes and dislikes in general.

If a spectacle frame is selected based upon above laws, it will fit comfortably, look good and will be used for a longer period of time to achieve the desired objectives. Based upon the laws of spectacle frame selection, it is, therefore, possible to devise a comprehensive guideline for various elements of spectacle frame as shown in Flowchart 4.2 that govern selection of an appropriate spectacle frame for a patient.

FRAME SIZE

The size of the frame is printed on the temples of the frame by the manufacturer. It is usually taken as horizontal distance between temporal outermost edges of an eyewire to its nasal outermost edge as shown in Figure 4.1. In a boxing system of measurement eyewire size is referred to as the "A" measurement. It is the widest horizontal measurement. Two eyewires

are connected with bridge width which is known as distance between lenses (DBL). Two eyewires and DBL taken together determines the total width of the spectacle frame front. In an ideal situation the total width of the frame front should be little larger than the facial width, so that it does not make contact at the temporal sides of the face. An ideal size of the frame follows the shape of the human skull without making any contact at the temporal sides. The straight forward meaning is the size of the frame selected should be in scale with the size of facial width as shown in Figure 4.2, and is fitted to ensure the philosophy of "the fitting triangle".

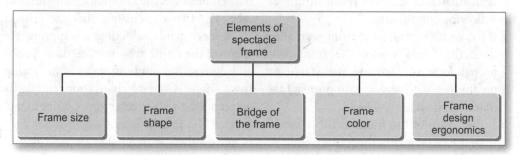

FLOWCHART 4.2: Elements of spectacle frame that govern frame selection

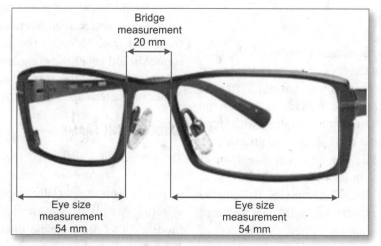

FIGURE 4.1: Frame size

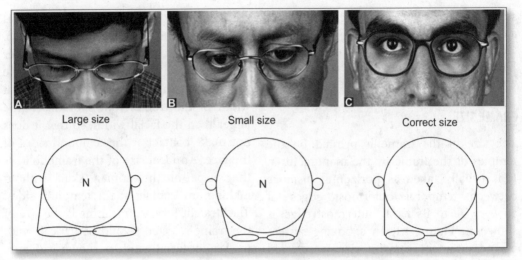

Large size   Small size   Correct size

FIGURE 4.2: Size of the frame with respect to facial width

A mismatch of size will result in one of the following conditions:
- If the width of the frame front is smaller than the facial width, the front will propel forward, denying the stable fit on the face and also creating unsightly marks at the temporal head.
- If the width of the frame front is larger than the facial width, the frame will have a tendency to slip down on the nose, making the overall fit loose.

FRAME SHAPE

Frames are exceedingly obvious on the face. The shapes of the frame may exaggerate and emphasize or disparage and deemphasize the facial characteristics. In an ideal situation the shape of the frame should contrast with facial shape, so that it can balance the proportion. Therefore, while selecting a suitable shape of the frame for an individual make sure that the selected shape maximizes the appeal of positive aspects of facial features and minimize the appeal of negative aspects of the face. The goal is to find a frame shape

that emphasizes the complimenting lines of face. The two dimensions that are critical to observe while selecting an appropriate shape of the frame are—vertical dimensions and horizontal dimensions of the frame front shape. General rule is longer face is better suited with greater vertical depth, i.e. greater "B" measurement and shorter face is more suited with smaller vertical depth, i.e. smaller "B" measurement. It implies that rectangular frame shape compliments better with round face, whereas aviator frame shape goes better with vertically oriented triangular face. Ideally, the shape of the frame should cover the eye adequately from all around, so that the eyes are at or near the center of the lens aperture of the frame.

BRIDGE OF THE FRAME

The essence of a well-fitted spectacle frame lies in the choice of appropriate bridge selection. This is specially important while selecting a plastic frame in which no modifications are possible once the lenses are fitted. The objective is to ensure even distribution of weight of the spectacle frame on a wider area of contact on the nose. Flowchart 4.3 shows the elements of bridge fitting, that are critical to observe while selecting a suitable bridge fitting for a plastic frame.

Width of the Bridge

Bridge width is the distance between lenses, it is the minimum horizontal distance between the nasal surfaces of the nasal rims in plastic or metal frames; or the minimum horizontal distance between the nasal edges of the lenses in the rimless frames (Fig. 4.3). Bridge width is responsible for correct frontal angle. Narrow bridge width may not be adequate to distribute the weight on the wider contact area, whereas wider bridge width may create additional weight on nose crest.

Base of the Bridge

Base of the bridge is the distance between the widest points of the bearing surface of

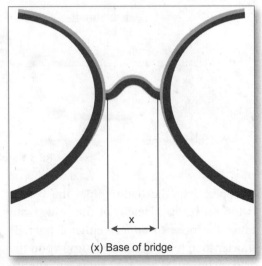

(x) Base of bridge

FIGURE 4.4: Base of the bridge

the bridge (Fig. 4.4). The base of the bridge should rest on the nose crest in case of plastic frames, whereas in metal frame it should not come in contact with the nose crest.

Height of the Bridge

Height of the bridge is the distance between the center of the bearing surface and the datum line, measured in a plane parallel with that of the frame front as shown in Figure 4.5. When the center of the bearing surface is in line with the datum line, the bridge is said to have "0" height. If the bridge surface is lower than the datum line, the bridge is down set bridge and if the bridge surface

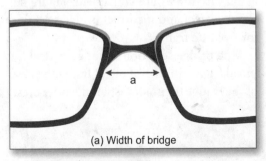

(a) Width of bridge

FIGURE 4.3: Width of the bridge

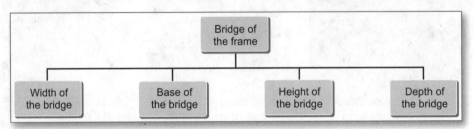

FLOWCHART 4.3: Important elements of bridge for frame selection

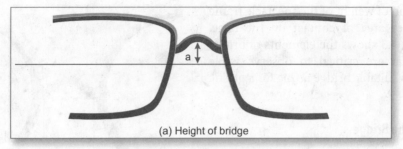

FIGURE 4.5: Height of the bridge

is upper than the datum line, the bridge is top set bridge. Height of the bridge can cause the nose to appear either longer or shorter than it really is, depending upon the bridge chosen. A top set bridge will expose the nose to appear longer than what it is, whereas a down set bridge will shorten the apparent length of the nose.

Depth of the Bridge

Depth of the bridge is the protrusion of the bridge, i.e. the bridge of the frame front is projected out as shown in Figure 4.6. More projection implies high depth of the bridge. Depth of the bridge is not as important fitting issue as it is the cosmetic issue.

Bridge is one of the most important elements for an ideal frame selection as far

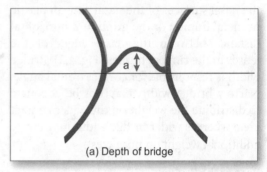

FIGURE 4.6: Depth of the bridge: distance between the center point of the bearing surface and a line representing the base of the bridge

as plastic frames are concerned. Figure 4.7 show correct and incorrect bridge selection for a plastic frame.

The bridge selection is not as critical for metal frame. In case of metal frame the base of the bridge does not rest on the nose crest.

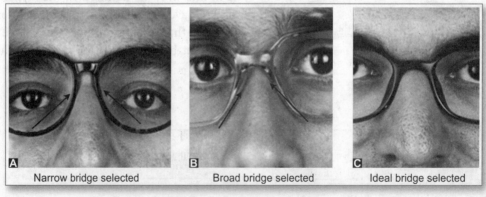

FIGURE 4.7: Different bridge fitting

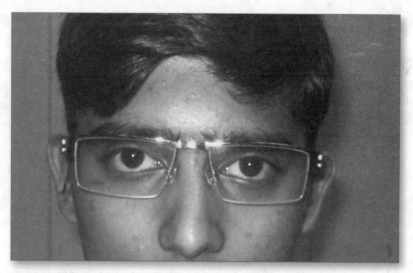

FIGURE 4.8: Bridge does not rest on the nose in case of metal frame

The entire weight of the spectacle frame rests on the flat surface of the pads as shown in Figure 4.8.

FRAME COLOR

Frame color selection depends upon the user's skin and hair color. Men usually look good in dark colors. Brown, black, gray and dark blue are popular color for men whereas red, pink and aqua are more popular in females. Females usually prefer lighter tones. Black is equally common for both specially young male and female.

Face color may be cool or warm. Cool color has blue or pink undertones whereas warm color has peaches or cream undertone or yellow cast. Everyone looks good in their own color tone. Frame color should complement facial color complexion. Colors may be solid or vertically gradient or horizontally gradient. Solid color has a shortening effect, i.e. the apparent length of the face seems shortened when you put on solid color frame. Gradient colors, specially vertically oriented gradient colors have a face lengthening effect, making them more compatible for wider face.

Occasionally, hair colors are also taken into consideration while selecting the frame color. Black, white and brown for hair color is taken as cool colors and golden and dirty gray is taken as warm color. Warmer color frames look good with golden hair. Pink tone best suits brown hair.

FRAME DESIGN ERGONOMICS

There are certain important elements of frame design that create the intended relationship between the structures of the frames and the wearers. They are engineered to maintain a balanced and secure fit, crafted to ensure comfortable contact at the bridge of the nose and behind the ears, and to provide an innovating new look to the overall design of the frame. The temples are attached to the extension of the front of the spectacle frame termed as lug. Temples are side bars that run from the joints across the sides of the

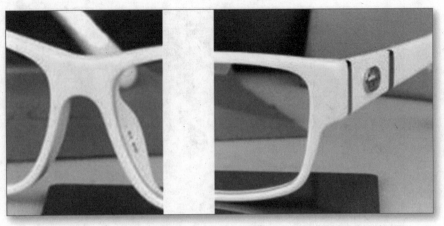

FIGURE 4.9: Top joint frames

head, thus holding the spectacle to the face. Temples interject an artificial dividing line that divides the frame front into two halves. The lower the line shorter the face appears and higher the line longer the face appears when viewed from the sides. If the temples are attached high on the frame front (Fig. 4.9), there is more facial area below the line and face appears lengthened. If the temples are attached lower on the frame, there is less distance from this line to the bottom of the chin and therefore, face appears shorter (Fig. 4.10). Temple thickness also affects the look of the facial length with broad temples reducing the apparent facial length and thinner temples increasing the apparent facial length.

The position of the joints in the vertical plane along the front also affects the fit of the frame. Low joint frames cause greater fitting problem than high joint frames because their center of gravity may result in somewhat precarious balance. Moreover low joints affect the inferior temporal field of view while high joints normally do not. A center joint temple may affect the temporal field of view. The angle of sides of low joint frames differs noticeably from other two types in that it usually has to have a negative value. Thus, it has a lot of

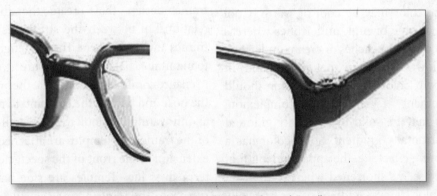

FIGURE 4.10: Temple joints little above datum line

impact on choice of the appropriate frame selection.

Bridge style can also be selected to hide the negative aspects of the nose. In order to lengthen the look of the nose, choose a frame that exposes as much of nose as possible. The keyhole bridge exposes most of the nose because it rests on the sides and not on the crest. To shorten the look of nose, choose a frame with a low or solid colored bridge and avoid a keyhole bridge, or a high bridge, or a clear bridge. To narrow and lengthen a wide nose use a clear or metal bridge that sits close to the nose and use nose pads on metal frames.

Frame selection entails more considerations than just understanding appropriate frame size, shape and other elements of frame fitting. An individual who is going to use the frame carries his own perception values and cosmetic considerations in addition to the healthcare issues that are generated because of lens prescription. It is also important to consider three factors as shown in the Flowchart 4.4, while selecting an appropriate spectacle frame for an individual.

LENS PRESCRIPTION

There are three important elements of lens prescription:
• Lens power
• Prescribed prism
• Pupillary distance.

Lens prescription influences all aspects of frame selection—size, shape, material and also frames styles. The general rule for frame selection is smaller size for prescriptions having high lens power. This is basically to reduce the lens mass and edge thickness in case of high minus prescription so that a cosmetically thin and light lens may be dispensed. This is also important to minimize the effect of oblique astigmatism. A symmetrical shape is more appropriate to ensure uniform thickness from all around in case of high minus lens prescription. Square, round or broader oval shape frames where the difference between "A" measurement and "B" measurement is relatively small are better than steep rectangular shape that creates a larger disparity in lens edge thickness in their horizontal meridian as compared to vertical meridian. High astigmatic lens should ideally be fitted in frames with sharp features and corners. A perfect round shape frame may not allow perfect axis orientation. Plastic material frames allow weight distribution on wider area of contact than the metal frames. Rimless frames are not good for high powered lenses for all the known reasons. Supra frames should not be considered for plus lenses, as thinner edge may not provide adequate groove width to fit the lenses.

For presbyopic prescription the frames must have sufficient depth or relatively larger "B" measurement to ensure adequate area for distance and near viewing zones. They should not reduce the size of the reading area by being too "cut away" in the nasal area of the frame. For example, aviator style frames

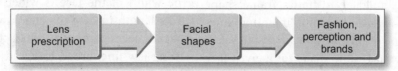

FLOWCHART 4.4: Factors that influence frame selection

may present such difficulties if coupled with narrow pupillary distance. Square and rectangular shapes are more suitable for all types of multifocal lenses which allow wider near zone to read through. Narrow oval shapes or steep rectangular shapes are not the ideal choice for multifocal lenses. Metal frames with adjustable nose pads allow flexibility of refinement of fitting even after fitting the lenses. They are, therefore better option for progressive addition lenses.

Pupillary distance measurement is also important criteria. The general rule is smaller frame size for narrow pupillary distance measurement and larger frame size for wider pupillary distance measurement. Shapes like square or rectangles are better options for prescribed prisms to prevent lens disorientation.

FACIAL SHAPES

There is nothing more important than how your eyewear looks on your face. A good looking frame makes the wearer feel good, sophisticated, polished, snazzy, attractive, stylish and confident. Theoretically, there are several factors that influence the frame selection, but in practice facial shapes dominate the most while selecting the appropriate frame shape. The shape of the frame should contrast with facial shape, so that it can balance the proportion. It should maximize the positive aspects of facial features and/or minimize the negative aspects of the face. The overall size of frame should be in scale with face size. The goal should be to find a frame shape that emphasizes the complimenting lines of face. One of the most ideal ways to select an appropriate frame shape for a given face is to analyze the face shape by comparing

the length of the face to its width. Then observe the bone structure and cheeks below the eyes and match the frame shape that emphasizes the complimenting lines of face. The following guidelines may help for different facial shapes:

Oval Face

Oval face is considered to be perfect ideal facial shape for most spectacle frame shapes. The perfect oval shape of the face has a length that is one and half times the width, with no obvious angles. Almost all types of frame shapes compliment with the oval shape face. The thumb rule while selecting the frame is "maintain oval's natural balance".

Round Face

Round face is characterized by almost similar proportion of length and width. In such case the shape of the frame should make the face look longer and thinner. Frame shape with wider "A" measurement than "B" measurement will create an effect that creates angles or horizontal lines and makes the facial shape appear longer and thinner. Rectangular shapes will be the most ideal that will cover the full facial width. Wider bridge will also add to size and clear bridge widens the look of eyes. Dark colored temples add width. Metal frame with rocking pads will keep away the lower rim from fuller cheeks.

Square Face

The width of the face is wider in relation to its length in case of square face. Square shaped faces are also characterized by strong jaw line, broad forehead and broad cheek bones and wide chin. The frame shape should make the face look longer. Select frame with weight on the top of the frame. This will give a look of lengthening the face. Oval shape frames with top or center joint will suit better. Decorations and dramatic designs at the upper temporal corner will lengthen the face. Narrow shape with larger "A" measurement will be better option.

Triangular Face

The face has wider forehead and higher cheek bones and narrow chin and jaw lines. The ideal selection of frame shape will draw the attention away from the forehead and will balance the narrow jaw with the frame shape. Taper shape from top, cat's eye shape or aviator shape frames may suit. Light and delicate styles are better. This is the difficult facial shape to select the frame for. Top heavy frame, i.e. thicker top rim or metal front with top plastic mount should be good.

Diamond Face

The diamond shaped face is the rarest face shape. The shape of face is narrow at the eye line and the jaw line with a small forehead and chin. Cheekbones are high and raised. The frame shape should widen the forehead and jaw and minimize the appearance of cheekbones. Choose frames that are heavy on top but avoid low temples joints frames. Rimless, square frames or straight top frames may work. Select square or straight top with bottom curved frames.

FASHION, PERCEPTION AND BRANDS

Spectacle frames are no more a mere necessity. They are also considered as precious luxury and ultra glamorous accessory that also make a fashion statement. Gone are the days when people used to wear anything as their eyeglasses so that they could see. Today spectacle frames are jewellery for eyes and are crafted by supremely creative and prodigiously talented designer and carry huge brand values. Brands like Cartier, Tiffany, Henri Julien, Daniel Swarovski, Bulgari, Prada and Mont Blanc all have opulent, breathtakingly beautiful precious eyewear frames and like all other stylish accessories, they also follow latest trends and styles in frames shape, styles and colors. Moreover, classy and stylish eyewear that find high favor with the celebrities also entice people to embrace. People who are entrapped by these perceptions are very conscious about their perceived ideas. They appreciate things that are different from normal and have character. They have their own opinion and DNA in whatever they attire. They look into themselves, the way they think and they try to make it mean something. The boundary of their thoughts is defined by them. The straight forward meaning is fashion and perception are complex area and when there is a question of fashion, perception and brands, no logic applies and no rule is followed.

Some people like to relate their eyewear to their mood and occasion. Understanding lifestyle need is the key to cater specific needs. For them one style is not for all occasion. They would appreciate to have their eyeglasses for every activity they participate in. They would like to appreciate classic style frames to present soft and streamlined look. Sometimes they would like to embrace creative styles frames that are more electrifying innovative and unusual while other time they would wear dramatic style frames having bold features and striking colors. Perhaps you need to be a good follower to talk in their language, not imposing your dispensing skills and ideas.

To sum up a basic guideline for ideal frame selection may be drawn as follows:

1. Know your facial features and facial contours: facial height to facial width ratio, bone structure and cheeks below the eyes.
2. Know your lens power and lens type.
3. Select a frame shape that contrasts with your facial shape to balance: maximizing the positive aspects and/or minimizing the negative aspects of your face.
4. Top edge of the frame front should not go higher than the line of your eyebrows and the lower edge of the frame front should not touch your cheeks, even while you smile.
5. Frame size should be in the scale with your facial width, i.e. outer edge of the frame front should not go beyond the temporal bone of your face.
6. Select the frame color that compliments your face complexion and hair colors.
7. Select a frame that exposes your nose as much as possible. A top bridge will expose the nose to appear longer than what it is.
8. Select frames that cater your perceived values.

Remember a good looking frame is also comfortable to wear. It makes the wearer feel good and comfortable. Wearing something that makes you feel good and comfortable gives you a nice perspective of the day ahead of you. Thus, buying the right frame will just be a breeze.

POINTS TO REMEMBER

- The size of the spectacle frame for an individual should be selected in scale with the size of the facial width.
- The shape of the frame for an individual should be in contrast with his facial shape.
- The correct selection of bridge is specially more important in plastic frame as no modification are possible once the lenses are fixed.
- Bridge width is responsible for correct frontal angle.
- The base of the bridge rests on the nose crest in case of plastic frame, but it does not rest on nose crest in case of metal frame.
- If the temples are attached high on the frame front, there is more facial area below the line and face appears lengthened.
- The general rule is smaller size for prescriptions having high power. This is basically to reduce the lens mass and edge thickness in case of high minus prescription, and lens mass and center thickness in high plus prescription.
- Oval shape face is the most ideal facial shape for spectacle frame.
- Rectangle shape frames are most ideal for round shape frames.
- A top bridge will expose the nose to appear longer than what it is.

LENS SELECTION

Lenses must suit the prescription, lenses must fit the frames, lenses must match the lifestyle, lenses must meet the visual demands and the lenses must ensure safety for the eyes. They are all important issues while selecting a suitable lens for a patient. Chapter 5 is designed to acquaint the reader with principles and theories that are applicable to achieve aforementioned objectives.

The changing visual needs of occupations and lifestyle have changed the way people use their eyes today. On the front of ophthalmic lenses too there have been a lot of development that have given several new types of ophthalmic lenses that vary widely in terms of material, design and application. Today's ophthalmic lenses are no more a piece of glass or plastic, they are highly technologically driven and they differ a lot with respect to their material composition and surface geometry. The straight forward meaning is that the selection of right lens for a patient is more difficult than ever before. There is a need for judicious application of optical intelligence to select a right lens together with psychological boosting of the patient not only to meet the unique visual needs but also to achieve four broad objectives of spectacle lens dispensing as shown in the Flowchart 5.1.

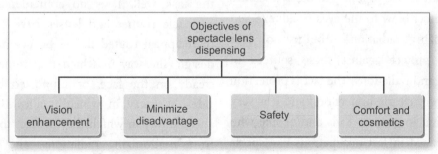

FLOWCHART 5.1: Objectives of lens selection

Vision Enhancement

Lenses are used to enhance vision and lenses are also used to maintain vision. This implies that there is a need for the best dispensing advice in terms of lenses to be used and surface treatments in the form of tints and coatings to be applied on lenses. Patient does not know what material the lens should be used or how they should be tinted or coated. It cannot be left entirely to their own discretion. Optician, taking care for these factors enjoys patient's loyalty that has positive impact on their practice.

Minimize Disadvantage

Disadvantages like poor fit, heavy lenses, steaming up, lens fogging, lens scratching, unsafe material and restricted field of clear vision should be minimized. This is an important aspect of dispensing for which professional advice is essential. The intended and unintended optical effects of lenses need to be explained to the patient to enable them to make an informed decision.

Safety

The main source of injury to the eyes comes from direct blow to the eyes or adnexa and nonionizing radiations. The use of lens should protect against these sources of trauma and radiations. The fact is protection is not very clearly understood and it is very important in general. Kids and people who are engaged in fast occupations like sports are highly susceptible to the sources of injury.

Comfort and Cosmetics

Comfort and good cosmetics are essential in lens dispensing. If a spectacle is uncomfortable, or cosmetically unacceptable—the danger of course is that it is not worn and the eye is not protected. It is important that the lenses do not make them feel out of date or conspicuous. A good looking spectacle makes the wearer feel good, sophisticated, polished, snazzy, attractive, and stylish and is also comfortable to wear.

FACTORS THAT AFFECT IDEAL LENS SELECTION

The ophthalmic lens dispensing is concerned about the real world and the practical difficulties of daily life. It is much beyond the boundaries of theories and principles of science. The optician cannot shelter behind the guidelines of science and absolve himself of the responsibility for the care of the patient. In terms of aesthetics, which reflects the wearer's desire to wear a vision-care solution, it is very important to understand that a mode of correction that is not looking good will detract him from the pleasure of wearing. Moreover, beautiful objects are often seen as if they also perform the task well. It is no coincidence that spectacle frames and lenses have part of their appeal routed in the beauty of their design; the way in which the frame stays steady on the face, or supported by the sides, the way in which it allows vision and the way in which they protect the eyes from nonionizing radiations. The art of dispensing is to provide maximum visual information. Patients do not know which lens material is right or what lens design will suit his prescription best or how they should be tinted or coated. It cannot be left to their own discretion only. The bottom line is it is the professional responsibility of the dispensing optician to provide his expert advice as to the lens selection and while doing so he must ensure that the lenses advised by him should meet four important objectives. While making an appropriate selection of lens for a patient the optician should consider three important factors as shown in the Flowchart 5.2.

Visual Needs

The need for visual correction is felt when an individual finds it difficult to meet his primary occupational visual needs. Occupational visual needs are nothing but the way an individual interacts with his visual environment. Immediate dissatisfaction is noted when a person's primary visual needs are compromised. It implies visual needs forms the basis for spectacle lenses and the only way to understand the visual need of an individual is getting into his lifestyle. The visual needs in occupations like surgeons, pilots and computer professionals are primarily near and extended near vision distance. Vision may be enhanced for near and extended near distance at the cost of long distance vision. Enhanced near vision lenses provide clear vision at near and extended near vision distance and at the same time minimizes the disadvantages of progressive addition lenses to provide the wider field of clear vision at intermediate distance. Half eye reading glasses works very well for avid readers. Direct blow and nonionizing radiations are two important safety issues in dynamic occupations like sports where the toughness of polycarbonate or trivex lens materials helps preventing trauma. Fixed and changing tints are used to prevent eye from the nonionizing radiations. Dark brown, dark gray or polarized lenses facilitate day driving. Amber yellow tints with antireflection coating works wonderfully during night driving.

Lens Prescription

The lens prescription is the reason for wearing the ophthalmic lenses. It is the first important factor that affects the selection of an ideal lens. Myopes are more benefitted by lens material whereas hyperopes are more benefitted by lens design. A high index lens material reduces the lens edge thickness and

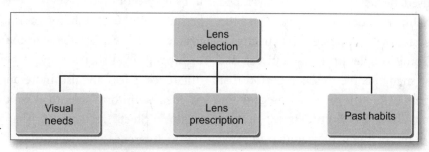

FLOWCHART 5.2: Factors affecting ideal lens selection

thereby reduces lens mass. When designed in aspheric lens form it also enhances the field of clear vision through the lenses and also adds cosmetic value to the lenses. An aspheric lens form will provide flatter look to a high plus lens prescription and thereby minimizes the lens bulge. When dispensed in high index lens material it also results in reduction of center thickness and lens mass. Organic plastic lens materials with antireflection coating are ideal lenses for low power prescription for safety, comfort and good vision. Cases like anisometropia are more benefitted by a judicial combination of lens material with different indices for right and left eye. The presbyopic list of lenses includes segmented multifocal and no-line progressive lenses, the choice between two broad category is mostly governed by factors other than the lens prescription.

Past Habits

There are several factors like physical, physiological and psychological that influence the ability of a person to see details. Over a period of time the person develops a habit that influences the visual system to see the details. Every time a new lens is used, he needs to break his developed visual habits to redevelop a new, to use the visual system with the new lens effectively. While some people are lucky and can see well, for many people this is a period that has to pass before they really appreciate the new lens. They take a little longer time to adapt. Some of them may notice unusual visual sensation during the adaptation

period. The straight forward implication is adaptation is easier and faster when changes are least. It is, therefore, important that while asking such patient to change the past habit with a new type of lens design, an informed choice is made and the patient is advised to spend a short period of time to adapt. The better the patient understands what he needs to do to adjust, the better are the chances of successful adaptation. Where the change involves single vision to bifocals or trifocals or the progressive lens, the patient should be given a balanced information about limitations and benefits of the lens type. Changing from one index material to another, from tinted lens to clear lens or vice-versa, wider segmented bifocals to progressive lens design—all of these cases needs good understanding of patient's visual needs. Care should be taken while changing the lens type when there is a great change in lens prescription. This is because in case of nonadaptation they invariably accuse the new lens type and blames the optician, leading to disappointments or anguish.

The shape, size, style and the material of selected frame also influence lens dispensing. The larger sizes of frames are not suitable for high power lens prescription because of the possibility of thicker and heavier lenses. Square shape or round shape or broader oval shape frames where frame difference is less are also more appropriate to ensure uniform lens thickness from all around. Steep rectangular shape where frame difference is large creates a disparity in lens edge thickness in their horizontal meridian as compared to vertical meridian. Plastic frames where overall weight of the spectacle is distributed on a wider contact area are more suitable for thicker lens power than the metal frames where the total weight of the spectacle frame is on two nose pads. Presbyopic lenses need larger "B" measurement to ensure adequate area for distance and near viewing zones. They should not reduce the size of the reading area by being too "cut away" in the nasal area of the frame. Square and rectangular shapes are more suitable for all types of multifocal lenses which allow wider near zone to read through.

MAKING AN IDEAL LENS SELECTION

The explosion in digital devices is all around us that have changed the "distance dominant world" to almost complete "near point world". There is a great change in how modern people respond to the changes in their visual demands. Many of them do not even know the modern solutions available to respond to these changing visual demands. Moreover, most patients do not know their own visual needs and the solutions available. They are guided by old perception that the spectacle lenses are used to see either at distance or at near. They cannot relate their occupational needs to visual needs. The patient who is looking for a solution considers the optician an expert lens consultant who will help him selecting a suitable frame and will advise an appropriate lens. Under such circumstances, it is the primary responsibility of the optician to discover the need and dispense suitable lenses that meet the primary objectives of

spectacle lens dispensing. The optician may pick up ideas from the medical practice wherein a medical practitioner makes diagnosis by asking relevant questions and then proposes appropriate solutions. In depth lifestyle questioning and listening may be very effective methods that can be applied effectively to understand visual demands of a patient that can create a strong foundation to make an ideal lens selection. Questions related to his lens prescription, his occupations, visual demands and lifestyle are important to elicit the criticalities of lens prescription and to get the desired information. Together with asking questions, equally important is intent listening. Most people do not listen with an intention of understanding; they listen with an intention to reply. In the process they miss lot of information. Patient listening, intent thinking and dynamic responses are important to successful lens dispensing. Every word spoken carries weight and meaning. The optician has to discover various visual needs and establish it as a point of concern for him and then advise suitable lens to align with discovered visual needs of the patient. It is wise to focus on his pain, and address the issue with the lens. This is possible only when the optician have comprehensive knowledge about two important attributes of lenses—lens design and lens material. All lenses differ either with respect to their material or design (Flowchart 5.3). It is important for the optician to know how he can improve the lens performance by selecting a correct blend of lens design and lens material for a patient.

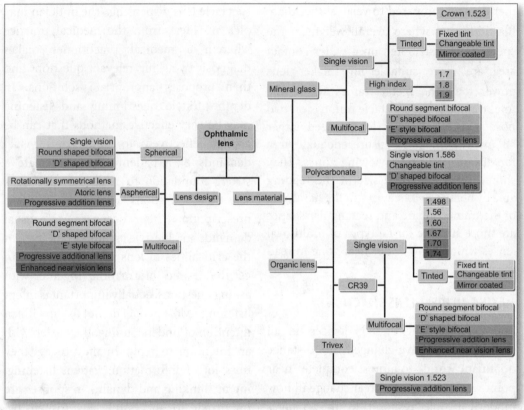

FLOWCHART 5.3: Lens map showing lens design and lens material

Lens Design

Lens design refers to the various lens forms that represent the shapes of two lens surfaces. The shapes of the two surfaces are determined by their curves which could be a single curve or multiple curves. Some of the examples of lens forms are: Bi-Cx, Bi-CC, meniscus, Plano-Cx, Plano-CC, spherical, aspheric, atorics, lenticular, or any other form that improves the optical performance of the lens. A complicated lens form may be defined in terms of mathematical equation.

When the lenses are designed with one single surface curve, it is known as spherical lens form. Spherical lens is a part of a sphere that is characterized by uniform radius of curvature in all the meridians from center to the periphery. Spherical lenses are designed based upon "best form lens design" philosophy. The best form lens is one that is designed to look good cosmetically and is also to minimize the effect of troublesome off-axis aberrations, i.e. it ensures a good balance between optics and cosmesis. Base curve selection forms the basis of spherical lens design. The unique features of spherical lens surface are:

- Spherical forms have higher sagittal height, resulting in high curve lens that magnifies or minifies the eyes and have more bulges when fitted in frame.
- Overall lens mass is more making the lens heavier and thicker.

- The peripheral lens portion results in an increased amount of oblique astigmatism that restricts the field of clear vision through the lens.

Most often lens designer deviates from the rule of "best form lens design" to make the lens look thinner and flatter. The result is observed as compromise in the lens performance. Flatter lens makes the lens look thinner, reduces lens mass and also enhances the cosmetic look of the lens, but at the same time degrades the off-axis visual performance of the lens because of increased oblique astigmatism. Contrarily, steeper lens provides wider field of clear vision because of reduced oblique astigmatism, but cosmetically they are unacceptable. The cosmetic benefit of flatter form was more acceptable than the optical benefits of the steeper lens form. The lens designer worked to minimize the effect of oblique astigmatism by introducing surface astigmatism. In the process they designed what is called aspheric lenses. The unique features of aspherical lens surface are:

- Aspheric lens surface is not perfectly spherical. At the center they are spherical but as you go towards the lens periphery, the surface power varies gradually in radial fashion, becoming progressively flatter or, steeper away from the center of the lens.
- The change in surface power is more noticed in the tangential plane of the lens than the change in sagittal plane. This difference in surface curvature produces surface astigmatism. The surface literally produces cylinder power away from its center that is used to neutralize the effect of oblique astigmatism produced by looking through the lens obliquely.

- As oblique astigmatism increases more and more while looking away from center in case of spherical lens design, asphericity changes more and more as you go away from its center.
- In case of plus lens the surface becomes flatter away from the center, if the asphericity is applied to the front surface of the lens, or the surface becomes steeper away from the center if it is applied to the back surface. In case of minus lenses the surface becomes steeper away from the center if asphericity is applied to the front surface of a minus lens, or the surface becomes flatter away from the center if it is applied to the back surface.

The rate of increase in surface astigmatism depends upon the degree of asphericity which is denoted by "e" value of the lenses. The "e" value defines the shape of the asphericity. Higher "e" value lens produces higher surface astigmatism. Since higher lens power produces higher oblique astigmatism, higher "e" value lens is needed to effectively increase the field of clear vision, whereas with low lens prescription smaller "e" value lenses may work. The underlying meaning is in an ideal situation aspheric lenses should be optimized for given lens power.

Like spherical lens surface aspheric lens surface is also designed based upon base curve selection. But it does not follow the guideline for base curve selection as given by "best form lens design" for spherical surface, instead a flatter base curve is being selected and the resultant effect of oblique astigmatism is offset by creating surface astigmatism. In addition to base curve, lens size also matters for degree of asphericity. Larger size lens needs high e-value lens than the smaller size.

Aspheric lens surface may be of following types:

- Rotationally symmetric asphericity
- Meridional asphericity
- Asymmetric asphericity.

Rotationally symmetrical aspheric lenses have been a very effective solution to minimize the effect of oblique astigmatism in case of higher spherical lens prescription. But the difficulties arise in case of sphero-cylinder lens prescription in which case meridional difference in power produces different oblique astigmatic effect in different meridians. A rotationally symmetrical lens surface in such case is compromised in one of the meridians. The lens designer, therefore, calculates different degree of asphericity for different meridians that improves the lens performance in terms of improving the overall field of clear vision throughout the lens surface. These lens surfaces are also known as "atoric lens". In case of atoric lenses the change in curvature away from the center varies from meridian to meridian. Asymmetric asphericity provides complicated lens geometry. Progressive addition lenses are asymmetric aspheric lenses.

The new free form process has totally changed the way the ophthalmic lenses are designed. You dream any form, you can design. The process is similar to lathe. The process of lens surfacing starts as a block of material. The block is cut using a single-point cutter that removes material from the spinning blank to create a desired surface. The cutter is precisely controlled by motors which follows a path contained in the form of a digital file. The resultant finished surface can be virtually any shape—with the potential for maximum precision. Free form process is a computer-based-numerically-controlled process that cuts the surface point by point, and thus can produce complex surface geometry. The process enables lenses to be produced to 0.01 D power accuracy and can reduce lens aberrations and yield less peripheral distortion and peripheral blur. Lenses can be customized to individual or personal specifications or preferences to improve the retinal image and thereby minimize any disadvantage; thus improving the visual performance of lenses on eyes. A new lens configuration can be designed that allows three-dimensional optical corrections, calculating the compensatory lens power in spherical, cylinder, axis and/or prism. The lens so generated may not match with the lens prescription, but provides the visual performance of the lens prescription in new configurations.

Lens Materials

Broadly, ophthalmic lenses are made of mineral materials or glasses and organic materials or plastics. In both categories there are several types of lens material available, each varying by their physical and optical properties. The correct selection of a lens material needs an in depth understanding of these properties which have a great impact on four important factors that govern the selection of lens material. These factors are shown in the Flowchart 5.4.

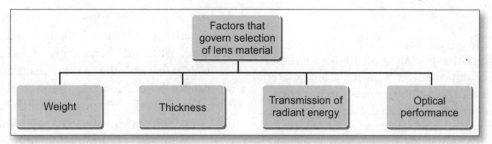

FLOWCHART 5.4: Factors that govern selection of lens material

Weight

The weight of a lens material is referenced by the term "density." or "specific gravity". Specific gravity of the lens material denotes the weight of the lens material in grams per cubic centimeter. Higher value of specific gravity indicates that the lens material is heavier and lower value of specific gravity indicates that the material is relatively lighter. A comparative study of density of various lens materials is shown in Table 5.1. Reduction of weight improves wearing comfort, and eliminates the indentations from nose pads that are produced by wearing heavy lenses. However, low density does not always mean a lighter spectacle—the lens mass is also an important criteria that ultimately depends upon the refractive index, lens size and the minimum thickness. Still it is one of the important factors for prescriptions that require high powered plus or minus lens prescription made in mineral glass lenses. Patients with high lens prescriptions are usually advised to use higher index lenses. Although they offer thinner lenses, they may not be more comfortable to wear because of their high specific gravity. A judicial approach while selecting the suitable lens material may compare the percentage gain in thickness reduction because of high index, vis-a-vis percentage increase in weight of the lens material.

Table 5.1:

Properties of lens materials				
Material	Index	Specific gravity (g/cm³)	Abbe value	Reflectance
CR 39	1.498	1.32	58	4.0
Poly	1.59	1.22	29	5.2
Trivex	1.53	1.11	46	4.4
Crown	1.523	2.54	59	4.3
1.60 Glass	1.60	2.60	42	5.3
1.70 Glass	1.70	3.20	35	6.7
1.80 Glass	1.80	3.66	25	8.2
Polyurethane	1.60	1.36	36	
High index plastic	1.694	1.41	36	

Thickness

The edge thickness of the minus lenses and the center thickness of the plus lenses are very important criteria for a lens material selection. As the lens prescription goes up, the thickness of both plus and minus lenses increases. The selection of an appropriate frame and an appropriate lens material can significantly reduce the final lens thickness, and thereby enhance the cosmetic look of the spectacle. The refractive index of the lens material determines its bending power and thus contributes to the lens power. A higher index of refraction results in a lower angle of refraction which means more light is bent for a given angle of incidence. This means higher refracting index lens materials have higher light bending power and lower refracting index lens materials have lower light bending power. The straight forward meaning is with higher index lens material, higher lens prescription can be made with less lens mass and flatter front and back curves. The end result we have a lens that is thinner than a lower index material.

Transmission of Radiant Energy

The electromagnetic spectrum is the distribution of electromagnetic radiation energy. The three regions of the electromagnetic spectrum are of prime concern when we talk about ophthalmic lenses:

- Visible light ranging from 380–760 nm is detected by human eyes.
- Ultraviolet (UV) ray is shorter than 380 nm.
- Infrared (IR) ray is longer than 760 nm.

As radiant energy passes through a lens, three possibilities are there, i.e. light transmission may be blocked, reduced, or not affected in these areas. UV rays are shorter wavelengths of light on the electromagnetic spectrum and they carry enough energy with them to damage ocular structure. Although human eye does not see UV radiation, the classic danger of UV cannot be overlooked. The protection from UV rays is only possible when the UV protection lenses are used as eyewears. Transmission of UV radiation through ophthalmic lenses may be reduced, blocked or not affected, depending on the lens material. It is important to understand how lens materials affect the transmission of UV radiation.

The IR rays lie at the longer wavelength part of electromagnetic spectrum beyond visible light. They produce thermal radiation and are not generally considered to be harmful to the eye as they carry low amount of energy. However, when the protection is desirable, the best protection from infrared rays is provided through metallic coatings on the lens surfaces that reflect the large amount of incident radiations. Dark green sunglass also absorbs IR radiations. Lens materials generally do not provide protection from infrared radiations.

Transmission of visible light can be affected by the color of a lens. White light is a combination of lights of different wavelengths in the visible spectrum. Passing white light through a prism splits it into the several colors of light observed in the visible spectrum. Transmission of visible light can be affected by the color of a lens material. Different colors can cause overall reduction or specific reduction in the visible region.

Optical Performance

The optical performance of any lens material is determined by V-value of the lens material and reflectance properties of the lens material. V-value or the Abbe number is the reciprocal of the dispersive power of the material. It measures the degree to which light is dispersed when entering a lens material. The lower the Abbe numbers the greater the dispersion of light causing the chromatic aberration in the periphery of the lens. The higher the Abbe number, the better the peripheral optics. Chromatic aberration is a type of lens aberration in which there is a failure of a lens to focus all colors or wavelengths of light to the same point. Chromatic aberration manifests itself as "fringes" of color along boundaries that separate dark and bright parts of the image. The common complaint is "the lenses are fine when I look through the centers but vision is blurred when look through the edge". When the wearer moves the eyes away from the center and looks through the periphery of the lens, the prism is created. The amount of prism created together with the dispersive value of the lens material, affects the amount of "color fringes" the wearer sees. BS 7394: Part 2, "specification for complete spectacles" classifies materials in terms of their Abbe number as follows:

- Low dispersion :$V \geq 45$
- Medium dispersion :$V \geq 39$ but < 45
- High dispersion :$V < 39$.

Abbe value is the property of the lens material and cannot be affected by lens designing.

Reflectance is another property that determines the optical performance of the lens material. It is the function of the refractive index of the lens. Reflection is more with higher index material. The phenomenon of light reflection occurs at each of the lens surfaces. The result is the loss of light transmission and undesirable reflections on the lens surfaces. The reflectance of the lens surface is material and design dependent. Higher index material and flatter lens surface increases loss of light because of surface reflection. The unwanted reflection can be almost completely eliminated by applying an efficient antireflection coating, the need of which is more in higher index material.

Based upon the fundamental rule that all myopes are most benefited by the lens materials and all hyperopes are most benefited by the lens design; a suitable lens can be selected by a judicious matching of lens material and lens design.

FUNCTIONAL CLASSIFICATION OF LENSES

A simplified functional classification of lenses categorizes the lenses with respect to their application and helps selecting the lenses for their function.

Driving Lenses

Driving is a high speed activity wherein our eyes work like a multitask performer—processing the speed and direction of other cars, recognizing signals and signs, spotting road hazards and identifying hairpin turns. Enhancing visual performance can really make driving a pleasant experience. Polaroid lenses can prevent glare and enhance visual performance to prevent eye fatigue during day driving. Light amber tint with antireflection coating prevents glare and minimizes the loss of light because of surface reflection for night driving. It also increases contrast. A dark tinted lens with back surface antireflection coating is useful for day driving. Photochromatic lenses that have ability to react to visible light or UV light are available in mineral glasses, plastic and polycarbonate material to provide one solution for day and night use.

Computer Lenses

Today computers are so much integral part of the life, that products used for computer related jobs have been named after the term "computer". In line with this researcher have developed the specially-designed lenses for computer purpose and they are being named as computer lenses. These lenses minimize the visual disadvantage during computer task and helps navigating the visual responses with ease. Visual fatigue is the biggest complain of the computer workers. Antifatigue lenses or stress relieving correction are one of the wonderful solutions for young computer workers. Presbyopes are more benefitted with refined near addition for computer monitor distance. Occupational enhanced near vision lenses are specially designed lenses; that meet the presbyopic demands of the patient's with extensive intermediate viewing needs. The lens design provides a reasonably large intermediate vision on the top of the lens to enable them to navigate the workplace. However, they do not meet general viewing needs outside the workplace. Glare and reflection are two important difficulties that computer user also face. Tints and antireflection coating may carry certain advantages for the computer.

Flat and Thin Lenses

The dispensing of flat and thin lenses is based on the cosmetic values. High index lens material provides thinner lenses that are very effective to minimize the lens mass and correspondingly lens weight. High index material dispensed in aspheric form, also makes the lens look flatter which is one of the most sought cosmetic advantage. They also result in reduced magnifications in high plus power and minifications in high minus lenses to add to the cosmetic values of the lenses. Aspheric lens also minimizes the effect of lens aberration that affects the off-axis performance of the lenses. They are also a great lens to reduce unwanted magnification and minification of your eyes.

Occupational Lens

Your visual skill controls visual performance, leading to occupational performance throughout your life. Occupational lens can be designed in single vision, bifocals or otherwise. Occupational enhanced near vision lenses and antifatigue lenses are newly designed occupational lenses that can be used for various occupation-specific purpose. The main objectives of dispensing occupational lenses are vision enhancement, minimizing disadvantage, protection from trauma and radiation, and comfort. Clip on lenses, billiards lenses, half eye spectacle, swimming glasses and sports lenses, are some other examples of occupational lenses.

Fashion Wear Lifestyle Lenses

Fashion wear lifestyle lenses are designed to cater fashion related aspirations of the wearer. One way mirror coating is applied on lens surface of clear or tinted lens to convert it into a lifestyle product. The mirror coating can be applied both in mineral glass and plastic. They are not only good to hide your eyes but also provide you high performance vision.

Life after 40 Lenses

Around the age of 40 years most patient starts having difficulties in near vision; signifying the onset of presbyopia. As the amplitude of accommodation diminishes, the range of clear vision may become inadequate for the patient's commonly performed tasks at several near or extended near distances. Thus, presbyopia is not just the problem of near vision at 40 cm, it is also a problem of reduced vision at various reading distances. Those who are involved more in near vision demanding tasks are likely to have more difficulty. Wide varieties of segmented and nonsegmented multifocal lenses are available in glass, plastic, polycarbonate and trivex materials. The endless menu of no-line multifocal lenses in all materials with fixed and variable tints to suit all your frames and avoid the discontinuities through bifocal and trifocal lenses are also available.

Reflection Free Lenses

Antireflection lenses are tuned to transmit 99% of available light. Superheated metallic oxides are applied on the lens surface permanently to create uniform filtering of light rays that optimizes contrast and minimizes reflection. The coatings are specially formulated for optical balance between reflection, transmission and absorption of light to enhance the visual performance.

Shatterproof Lenses

Organic plastic lens material offers superior comfort, clarity and protects against impact with greatest hit and UV radiations. Polycarbonate and trivex lenses are specially suited for kids and rimless frames. The toughness of poly lenses is tested against highest velocity and high mass impact.

DISPENSING HIGH-INDEX LENSES

BS 7394 Part 2 "specification for complete spectacles" classifies materials in terms of refractive index as follows:
- Normal index: $n \geq 1.48$ but < 1.54
- Mid-index $n \geq 1.54$ but < 1.64
- High-index $n \geq 1.64$ but < 1.74
- Very high-index $n \geq 1.74$.

Refractive index is the physical property of the lens material. It determines the light bending ability of the lens material. Higher refractive index implies that the light bending ability of the lens material is higher and consequently the need for the surface power is significantly minimized for a given lens power. The result is noted as reduction in edge thickness in minus lens prescription and center thickness in plus lens prescription. Several refractive indices of lens material are available ranging from normal to very high, the objective for each one is to reduce lens thickness and improve the cosmetic appeal of the lenses. The surface power of the lens is given by curve variation factor (CVF). CVF shows the variation in surface power when the lens material selected is other than standard crown or CR 39 lens material. It is a useful factor to know the likely change in the volume and thickness of lenses that will be obtained when another material is compared with the standard lens material. The CVF for different lens material as represented by their index of refraction are shown in Table 5.2.

Table 5.2:

CVF for different refractive indices		
Refractive index	*CVF*	*Specific gravity (g/cm³)*
1.523	1.00 D	2.54
1.70	0.75 D	3.20
1.80	0.65 D	3.66
1.90	0.58 D	4.02

Based upon values given in Table 5.2, if crown glass material is used for a lens power of –8.00 D, the algebraic summation of two surface power of the lens is also –8.00 D, whereas the surface power is reduced to –6.00 D when the refractive index of the material is changed to 1.70 and is further reduced to –5.20 D and –4.64 D when the refractive indices used are 1.80 and 1.90 respectively. Using resultant surface power, the center and edge thickness can be calculated which may be used to compare the percentage gain in lens thickness that can be achieved by using higher refractive index lens material. However, higher refractive index lens materials also have higher specific gravity that may lead to increase in lens material weight. It is, therefore, prudent to compare the percentage gain in lens thickness against the percentage increase in lens weight to make a correct selection of suitable material. This may not be an important factor for organic lens material, but this is very important criteria for mineral lenses. The important point to note here is that the overall weight of the spectacle is the function of several factors, not just the refractive index of the lens material. The overall weight of the spectacle can also be reduced by:

- Selecting a smaller size frame.
- Distributing the overall weight on the wider area of contact on the nose.
- Selecting light-weight frames.

An ideal situation for high-index lens dispensing includes:

- Select a lens material with an appropriate index with respect to lens prescription. A good approach may be very high-index lens material for very high lens prescription and a mid-index lens material for low to moderate lens prescription.
- Select a smaller size frame with symmetrical shape.
- Select a frame that is made of plastic frame with saddle bridge.
- Select a light weight frame.

In addition, while dispensing high-index lenses following additional care must be taken:

1. Do not jump into selecting a very high-index lens material for low to moderate lens prescription because most high-index lens materials have lower Abbe value, which means optical performance of the lens material is compromised from the lens peripheral portion. Higher-index lens material causes greater dispersion of light, causing more chromatic aberration in the periphery of the lens. Chromatic aberration is a type of lens aberration in which there is a failure of a lens to

focus all colors or wavelengths of light to the same point. Chromatic aberration manifests itself as "fringes" of color along boundaries that separate dark and bright parts of the image. The common complaint is: "The lenses are fine when I look through the center but vision is blurred when I look through the edges." Higher the index, higher is the error. The effect of chromatic aberration can be controlled by a judicious selection of correct index of lens material and also by carefully placing the optical center and dispensing the smaller size frames.

2. Higher refractive index also results in increase in surface reflection of light. Surface reflection reduces the light transmission through the lens and results in poor visual performance. However, loss of light because of surface reflection can be very well minimized by applying antireflection coating on the lens surface. In fact all high-index lenses should always be dispensed with antireflection coating.

3. The selection of base curve also needs to be compensated for the refractive index of the lens material. Base curve is selected with respect to the resultant surface power.

The current trend of dispensing high-index lens material with aspheric lens design makes the lens look flatter and thinner, that further enhances the cosmetic value. But care must be taken to dispense those lenses with antireflection coating as flatter surface also increases surface reflection.

DISPENSING TINTED LENSES

Tinted lenses are made to absorb the visible light and thereby reduce the light transmission. They are mostly dispensed to protect the eyes from the harsh luminous radiation. Tints may be fixed or variable. Variable tint darkens when exposed to UV rays. Light transmission level of tinted lens is specified in terms of luminous transmission factor (LTF or LT) as a percentage of light transmitted. For example, LT 80% brown tint transmits 80% of light averaged over the visible spectrum and absorbs 20%. Tinted lenses are most often dispensed for the following reasons:

1. Cosmetic reasons are one of the driving factors for dispensing tinted lenses because tints tend to complement skin tones and also remove some of the glassiness of the lenses.

2. If a patient has been comfortably using tinted lenses and is also fascinated to use the tinted lenses, it is prudent not to remove the tint for arbitrary reasons.

3. Patients with light pigmented iris or patients who are not in good health or patients who have neurological disturbances most often find themselves happier with tinted lenses.

4. Light sensitive patients are also benefitted with tinted lenses. Some of the common symptoms of light sensitivity is rapid blinking, poor concentration, lowering of chin to shield the eyes, narrowing of the palpebral aperture and epiphora.

5. Tints that lie at or beyond the peak spectral range are most often used as contrast enhancers. Night drivers are most benefitted with amber or orange tint with antireflection coating.

6. Sometimes tints are also used to enhance reading comfort and performance.

The visible light spectrum extends from about 380 to 780 nm that gives rise to light sensation. Different wavelength of light is perceived as different colors. Table 5.3 shows that different wavelengths of light associated with different color sensation.

Table 5.3

Color sensations associated with different wavelength of light	
Violet	400–420 nm
Indigo	420–440 nm
Blue	440–490 nm
Green	490–570 nm
Yellow	570–585 nm
Orange	585–620 nm
Red	620–780 nm

Based upon their wavelength values they provide different advantages to the wearer.

Violet

Violet tint is at the shorter wavelength end of the visible spectrum and is the immediate neighbor of UV rays and therefore it is always likely to carry UV with itself. It is, therefore, not an advisable tint for outdoor use. It is one of the least popular colors in dispensing optics.

Indigo

Indigo projects a compassionate nature. It is at shorter wavelength end of the visible spectrum and therefore, diminishes contrast. It is also one of the least popular colors in dispensing optics.

Blue

The element that is used to produce blue tint is cobalt. Blue transmits blue and UV rays and absorbs yellow and orange. It is also not recommended for outdoor use.

Green

The element that is used to produce green tint is iron. It absorbs blue and violet rays. It is also good for UV and IR protections. It acts as contrast enhancer and provides true color perception. It is a good tint to be used to minimize eyes strain and glare.

Yellow

The element that is used to produce yellow tint is uranium. It absorbs blue, violet and UV light. It lies at the peak spectral acuity and therefore makes everything brighter. Although it is a contrast enhancer, it disturbs color perception. It is good for occupations like shooting, snow skiing and hunting. But the use of yellow tint should be avoided directly under bright sunlight.

Orange

Orange tint is also a contrast enhancer, makes everything brighter. Light orange works wonderfully for night driving if it is used with antireflection coating.

Red

The element that is used to produce red tint is gold. Red blocks blue and blue-green wavelength. It is a contrast enhancer and is therefore good for skiing and hunting.

Brown

Brown is general purpose filter. It absorbs UV and also enhances contrast. It is very good for day driving.

Gray

Gray is a neutral density filter. It is good for light sensitive people and also for jobs which requires accurate color discrimination.

Tints are often prescribed on the preference of the wearer. What one believes is restful color, another may find it stimulating. Fashion tints need only the correct appearance, but special purpose tints should have a method of determination in terms of transmission and absorption as well as clinical judgment. There is a need for clinical test so that it can be used as a diagnostic tool to prescribe the suitable tint. However, in the absence any clinical tests tints may be based upon the following factors:

1. Luminous transmission factor
2. Light sensitivity
3. Contrast enhancement
4. Reduced migraine
5. Reading comfort and performance
6. Driving factor
7. Enhancement and protection factor.

Different lens material responds differently to the tints. Glass lenses are tinted by adding various oxides to the batch materials to give the lens a specific color. By adding the various metallic oxides to the glass constituents, the light absorption can be increased in almost any desired way, both within and beyond the visible spectrum. However, when there is a change in density across the lens surface due to the change in thickness from center to edge, the depth of tints may vary. It is for this reason minus glass tinted lenses show light tints at the center than the lens periphery and plus glass tinted lenses show darker tints at the center than the lens periphery. Plastic or organic lens material can be tinted by immersing in a container of dye. The dye is heated in a container and the lenses are immersed into the heated liquid to apply surface tint. The longer the lenses remain in the dye, the darker the tint is achieved. Interesting tint combination can be created to an individual's imagination. Graduated and double graduated effects are comparatively easy to achieve with the aid of a pulley mechanism which gradually lifts the lenses out of the tint tank, thus imparting more tint on one part of the lens than the others. One thing must be kept in the mind that it is difficult to predict how a pair of lens will react when immersed into a tint bath. Even though both the lens may be of the same material and also from the same manufacturer, the "take up" rate between the right and the left lens may be different. This can be due to a number of factors. One reason could be that one lens has been in storage for longer period than the other and thereby react differently when immersed into the tint bath. To reduce such problems always try to ensure that same manufacturer's lenses are tinted together, and both the lenses must be of the same index because higher index resin materials exhibit different characteristics that prevent them from being tinted to the darker shades. In case of plastic lenses tints may be removed and the lens may be tinted to give the effect of new color. Both glass and plastic lenses can also be mirror coated. A mirror coating can be applied by a vacuum process to the front surface of the lens causing the lens to have the same properties as a two way mirror. The observer, unable to see the wearer's eyes, sees his own image reflected from the lens. The wearer is able to look through the lens normally. There is, of course, a reduction in the transmission of the light because of the high percentage of light is being reflected. Mirror coatings are often used in combination with a tinted lens to provide more protection from intense sunlight. Mirror coating may be full, i.e. uniform throughout the lens surface or it may be graduated. Mirror coated lenses work by reflecting back specific wavelengths, whereas solid tints work by absorbing the wavelengths or light energy. Light energy absorbed expresses itself in the form of heat which might irradiate the eyes. But this does not occur in case of mirror coated tints as the energy is reflected away. The wearer also gets the benefits because the depth of the tint is uniform over the whole lens area irrespective of lens power and lens thickness.

DISPENSING LENSES FOR WRAP SPORTS FRAMES

The introduction of wrap sports frames requiring wrap around prescription lenses has given rise to some challenging and very unique ophthalmic fitting and lens power issues. Until recently, lenses for wrap frames have been made by producing the patient's prescription using high spherical base lenses which typically had a nominal front curve of 9 base. 9 base lenses are designed to fit the lenses into highly curved frame front to ensure the streamlined good looks of the wrap wear frames. In the process they violate the "best form lens design", creating unwanted power and prismatic error and the results are seen as patients having discomfort and nontolerance to adapt to lenses.

Look at Figure 5.1 wrap sports frames differs from dress wear frames as they have larger "A" measurement than "B" measurement and fits closer to the eyes. When fitted on face they demonstrate following unique features as shown in Table 5.4.

The new configuration of the fitting implies that the wearer is now looking through the lens on a different optical axis corresponding to the wrapped positioning as shown in Figure 5.2. The increased panoramic angle tilts the lens along the vertical axis and creates asymmetry between the nasal and temporal sides of the lens. The result is seen in the form of power error and astigmatic error across the entire lens surface. Prism error is also created due to

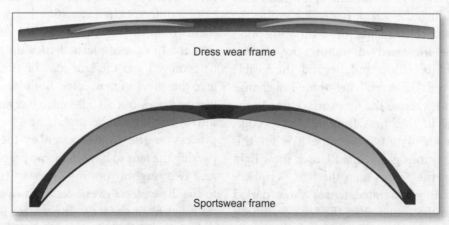

Dress wear frame

Sportswear frame

FIGURE 5.1: Sports wear frame and dress wear frame

Table 5.4:

A comparative features of sportswear frame fitting vs dress wear frame fitting		
	Wrap sports frame	*Dress wear frame*
Panoramic angle	15°–20°	4°– 6°
Pantoscopic angle	8°–10°	4°–6°
Vertex fitting distance	10–12 mm	14–16 mm

the angle between the line of vision and the lens optical axis. Increased pantoscopic angle tilts the lens around the horizontal axis that also results in power error and astigmatic error across the entire lens surface. The frame occupies a position such that the center of the pupil lies much above the horizontal center line, resulting in base down prism. Most wrap sports frame also fits closer to the eyes, which means refracted distance is greater than the fitted distance. The change in vertex distance causes change in effective lens power that can be calculated with the help of effective lens power formula. The overall result is noticed across the entire lens surface as:

• Induced unwanted prism
• Induced radial astigmatism
• Induced blur.

The patient finds a great deal of changes in the lens performance for central and peripheral power. The greater the degree of the wrap angle of the frame the greater is the effect. This is due to inadequate considerations being given to the need to re-calculate lens powers because of the optical effects associated with large amounts of panoramic and pantoscopic tilt in wrap frames. Lens power needs to be compensated for the changed configurations. The compensatory prescription is designed to calculate the new lens power so that the visual performance of the lens can be improved in wrap configurations that will provide visual clarity at all angles of view even at the edge of the lens.

Dispensing of sports lenses require certain additional dispensing measurements

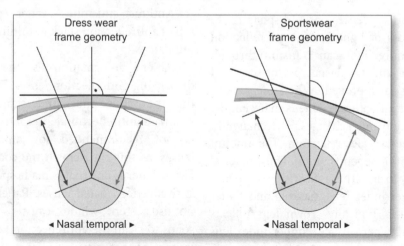

FIGURE 5.2: Effect of sportswear frame geometry

that need to be supplied to the lens laboratory. Some of the important measurements are:

1. Prescription (spherical, cylindrical, axis and prism).
2. Monocular pupillary distance measurement.
3. Vertical height measurements of optical center position.
4. Base curve of demo lens.
5. Frame eye shape and size.
6. Frame bridge size.
7. Horizontal inclination of the frame or dihedral angle.
8. Vertical inclination of the frame or pantoscopic angle.
9. Vertex distance measurement.

The above information is inserted into the sports lens software which calculates an aberration corrected lens power and optimizes the data to provide wider peripheral field of view and clear vision throughout the lens size. The lens is customized not only to frame but also to position of wear.

DISPENSING ANTIREFLECTION COATED LENSES

Antireflection lenses are dispensed to prevent loss of light because of reflection so that more light can transmit through the lenses and the visual performance of the lenses is improved. When the rays of light enter an ophthalmic lens material, the speed of light rays changes. The change in light's speed creates reflection. The amount of reflection depends upon lens material and lens form. The reflection is greater with higher-index lens material and flatter form lenses. Typically crown lens reflects light by 4.2% per surface. Higher-index lens material reflects upto 12–14% depending upon refractive index of the material. The refractive index of the lens material also influences the background color produced by antireflection coating. A similar effect occurs in case of organic plastic lenses where a front side semifinished hard coated lens is used. The result may be seen as difference between background color between front and back surface of the lenses. It means following care is very critical for dispensing antireflection lenses:

Avoid dispensing one lens at a time. Do not dispense one antireflection lens from ready stock series and other from prescription category. There is a possibility of mismatch of background color and coating affectivity. The difference in color has no effect on vision but is always noticed by the patient. Therefore, both the right and left lenses should always be made together.

Another typical issue with antireflection lenses is lower reflection of light implies that dirt and surface defects are more visible and it is difficult to keep the lens looking clean. Therefore, while dispensing antireflection lenses, look at following additional enhancement coatings like:

Antidust, antismudge, water repellent on top of antireflection stack to minimize these difficulties.

Patient information is the key to dispensing antireflection lenses. Make sure that the patient must understand how to maintain antireflection lenses. Dry cleaning is not recommended for antireflection lenses, as this can scratch the coating. The best cleaner is one that is made specially for antireflection coated lenses. Patient should not use acetone, windex, caustic solution or soaps to clean the antireflection lenses. It is important that every eyewear patient going through the office gets an explanation and demonstration of antireflection coating's benefits. This ensures that every patient understands you are trained and skilled in dispensing what has been accepted as the most advanced modern lenses available.

DISPENSING ASPHERIC LENSES

Aspheric lenses differ from spherical lens form in terms of their sagittal value and lens form. Aspheric lenses are flatter form of lenses (Fig. 5.3). Flattening a spherical lens surface introduces astigmatic and power error in the lens peripheral portion. Therefore, the peripheral curvature of the aspheric lenses has to change in a manner that neutralizes this effect, which is achieved by altering the peripheral curves of the lens surface. In plus lenses this is achieved by flattening the front aspheric surface or by steepening the back aspheric surface to reduce the effective gain in oblique astigmatic error; and in minus lenses this is achieved by steepening the front aspheric surface or by flattening the back aspheric surface to reduce the effective gain in oblique astigmatic error. The lens surface so designed shows the surface astigmatism. The objective of surface astigmatism is to neutralize the oblique astigmatism, produced when the wearer looks away from the center of the lenses. The amount of oblique astigmatism produced by a lens depends upon lens power. Therefore, the degree of asphericity should be selected based upon lens power. The degree of asphericity is denoted by "e" value of the lenses. Higher "e" value lenses have higher degree of asphericity and are more suitable for higher lens power. Since higher lens power creates higher oblique astigmatism; higher "e" value lens is needed to increase the field of clear vision effectively, whereas with low lens prescription smaller "e" value lenses may work. Therefore, in an ideal situation aspheric lenses should be optimized for given lens power.

Like spherical lens design an appropriate selection of base curve is equally important for aspheric lenses. But the selection of base curve does not follow the rule of "best form lens design". A flatter base curve is selected and degree of asphericity is designed to neutralize the effect of resultant oblique astigmatism. It is interesting to note that the flatter geometry of aspheric surface also reduces lens thickness. This is because of the fact that the sag of an aspheric surface is shallower than that of the spherical surface for a given lens diameter.

Fitting of aspheric lenses is somewhat similar to the way progressive lenses are

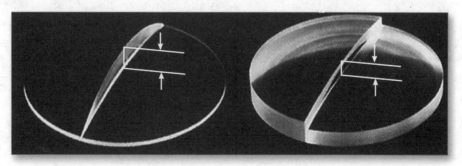

FIGURE 5.3: Aspheric lens surface geometry

fitted. Precise monocular pupillary distance measurement is essential to place the pole of the lens in front of pupil. Mark the vertical height of each pupil center on the lens insert of the frame, or it may be measured with reference to lower eye rim or datum line of the frame. The optical center should be lowered by 1 mm for every additional 2° of pantoscopic tilt (Fig. 5.4). However, the maximum drop should not be more than 5 mm. This is important to achieve the optical benefits of aspheric lenses in true sense which is possible only when the pupillary distance measurement of the patient is in alignment with geometric center or pole of the aspheric lens surface. This aligns the lens design rotationally around the optical axis.

The need for accurate placement of optical center of the aspheric lens throws up an issue on dispensing aspheric lenses for prescribed prism. Shifting of optical center to create prism will move the geometric center of the lens away from the optical axis of the eye which will cause unwanted visual disturbances for the patient because of non-alignment of pole with patient's pupillary distance. The straight forward meaning is prism by decentration is not recommended for aspheric lenses. Prescribed prism needs to be surfaced or worked to maintain the alignment of the aspheric geometrical center with the pupil and also have prism in the lens. In such case, the lens will have asphericity on front side of the lenses and the prism and cylinder at the back surface of the lenses.

Aspheric flatter lenses increases the loss of light because of surface reflection, hence all aspheric lenses should ideally be dispensed with antireflection coating. Flatter lens may also cause "lash crash" on the backside of the lens, where the patient's lashes brush against the lens surface. A concave curve on the backside helps position the lens further from the eye. Finally, some sensitive patients may notice that things look different with their new aspheric lenses. This is because aspherics lenses reduce magnification or minification upto 20% of normal size. This implies, there is a need to assure the patient that this is a positive change—their eyes will ease and enjoy the new view in just a few days.

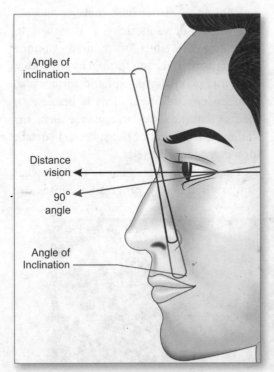

FIGURE 5.4: Dispensing aspheric lenses

POINTS TO REMEMBER

- The shape, size, frame style and materials—all influence the correct selection of a lens type.

- The appropriate selection of lens entails correct blend of lens material and lens design for a patient.
- A best form lens is one that ensures a good balance between optics of the lens and its cosmetic appeal.
- Larger lens size needs a high e-value aspheric lens surface.
- The edge thickness of minus lenses and center thickness of plus lenses are very important criteria for an appropriate lens material selection.
- The optical performance of any lens material is determined by V-value of the lens material and reflectance properties of the lens material.
- Myopes are most benefitted by lens material and hyperopes are most benefitted by lens design.
- The Abbe number of an ophthalmic lens material represents the relative degree of distortions generated while looking through the off-center areas of lens.
- Higher specific gravity denotes that the lens material is relatively heavier.
- Chromatic aberration results from the dispersive power of a material.
- Refractive index is the physical property of the lens material. Higher refractive index implies that the light bending ability of the lens material is higher.
- Tinted lenses are used to reduce the light transmission through the lens material.
- The tinted high minus glass lenses will have a lighter central portion, darkening gradually towards the periphery in glass.
- The tinted high plus glass lenses show a darkened central zone with the tint gradually lightening towards the lens periphery.
- Lens power needs to be recalculated and compensated for wrap configurations of frames to improve lens performance for central and peripheral visual performance of the lenses.
- The visual benefit that comes from increasing light transmission with antireflection coating is wearers see everything brighter and clearer with crisper details.
- An aspheric surface is a surface that is not perfectly spherical. It becomes progressively flatter or steeper away from the center of the lens.
- Aspheric lens works to counteract the positive oblique astigmatism arising from off-axis gaze by creating negative surface astigmatism. The negative surface astigmatism increases progressively as we move away from the vertex or pole of the aspherical surface.
- The sag of the aspheric lens surface is less than the sag of a spherical surface of the same radius.
- Aspheric lens is not being decentered to produce prismatic effect because the decentration will shift the pole of the surface from the visual axis.

PUPILLARY DISTANCE MEASUREMENTS AND OPTICAL CENTER OF LENS

There are some basic measuring skills, which are very critical in order to master the art of optical dispensing. Pupillary distance measurement is one of the most important of all. Measuring pupillary distance also necessitates learning the application of specially designed equipments that are used for the purpose. The objective of Chapter 6 is to elaborate the complete procedure for measuring interpupillary distance (IPD), applications of instruments and tools used for the purpose and dispensing the lenses to place the optical center of the lens in accordance with the measured pupillary distance.

Pupillary distance is the measure of distance between the center of the pupil of one eye to the center of the pupil of the other eye as shown in Figure 6.1.

It can also be measured from outer limbus edge of one eye to the inner limbus edge of other eye as shown in Figure 6.2.

Since pupil is displaced 0.3 mm nasally, limbal measure will be approximately 0.5 mm greater than the measure found using pupil center. The measurement of pupillary distance varies with the gaze angle of the patient. When a person looks at closer distance, his eyes turn in towards each other. As he lifts his eyes to look at longer distance the two eyes move away from each other. Pupillary distance for distance vision is measured when the patient looks in the straight ahead gaze direction when the eyes look at infinity and pupillary distance for near viewing gaze is measured when the patient looks at a distance of 40 cm. For this reason IPD for distance viewing angle is larger than IPD for near viewing angle. The amount of difference may vary between 4 and 5 mm. The measurement of IPD also varies because of age, but once a patient attains adulthood the measurement of IPD does not change. IPD determines the lateral or horizontal placement of the optical center of the spectacle lens. When the spectacle lenses are fitted into the spectacle frame, the distance between the optical centers of the

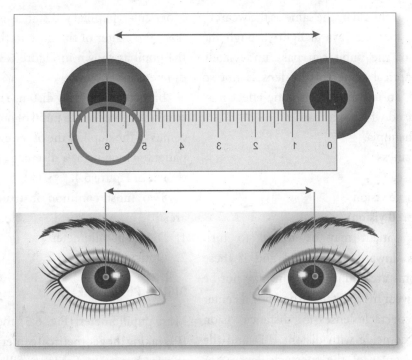

FIGURE 6.1: Anatomical IPD

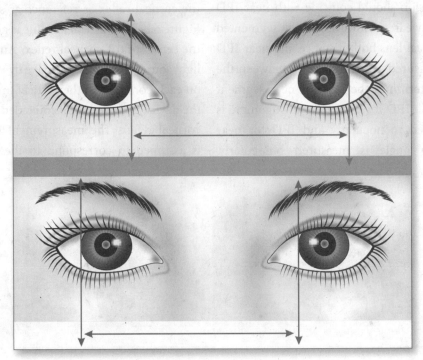

FIGURE 6.2: Measuring IPD from limbus to limbus

two lenses should be the same as the wearer's IPD, so that the rays of light through the center of the pupil can pass undeviated. If the optical center of the lens is not so aligned, an unwanted prismatic effect may be induced which may cause:

- Asthenopia
- Dizziness
- Nausea
- Double vision
- Blurred vision.

The patient may be forced to turn his eyes inward or outward and if these symptoms are bad, the person may not be able to wear his spectacle. The optical center of the spectacle lenses for distance vision should coincide with distant IPD and the optical center of the spectacle lenses for near vision should coincide with near IPD of the wearer. However, for a segmented multifocal lens both distance and near IPD are measured as the difference between the two determines the inset of near segment position. IPD for distance viewing angle is measured monocularly and IPD for near viewing angle is measured binocularly.

Monocular pupillary distance is measured from the center of the nose to the center of the pupil as shown in Figure 6.3. It may be different for two eyes.

Binocular pupillary distance is measured from the center of the pupil of one eye to the center of the pupil of the other eye when the patient is looking at a distance of 40 cms as shown in Figure 6.4.

Two most common instruments used are:

1. Digital pupillometer
2. Optician's ruler.

DIGITAL PUPILLOMETER

Most pupillometer (Fig. 6.5) measures the IPD taking the geometrical center of the pupil as reference point. Essilor pupillometer uses the corneal reflex as reference as shown in Figure 6.6. The vertical hairline is aligned to the center of the corneal reflex. An internal light source produces an image by reflection on each cornea, and the vertical line within the device is moved until coincided with the corneal reflex. The measurement so taken is assumed to correspond to the subject's

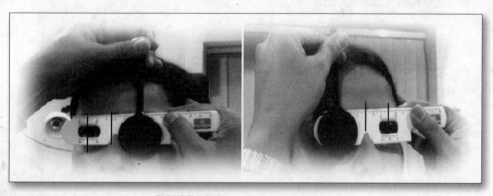

FIGURE 6.3: Measuring monocular PD

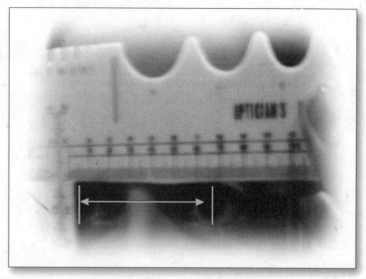

FIGURE 6.4: Binocular PD measurement

line of sight. The line of sight is defined as a line passing through the center of the pupil to the object of regard. This is the line that desirably passes through the optical center

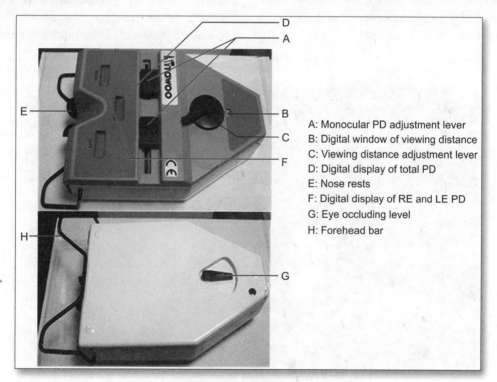

A: Monocular PD adjustment lever
B: Digital window of viewing distance
C: Viewing distance adjustment lever
D: Digital display of total PD
E: Nose rests
F: Digital display of RE and LE PD
G: Eye occluding level
H: Forehead bar

FIGURE 6.5: Pupillometer

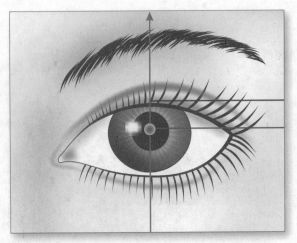

FIGURE 6.6: Corneal reflex alignment with vertical line

of the lenses and is the basis upon which the measurement of IPD rests. The advantage of using pupillometer is the measurements taken are not subject to parallax errors. Most pupilometer measuring range is 48–77 mm and the viewing distance is from 35 cm to infinity.

The sequential procedure of using pupillometer is as under:
1. Dispenser and the patient should be at the same level as shown in the Figure 6.7.
2. Take distance IPD monocularly and near IPD binocularly. Set the viewing distance 40–50 cm for near PD measurement and

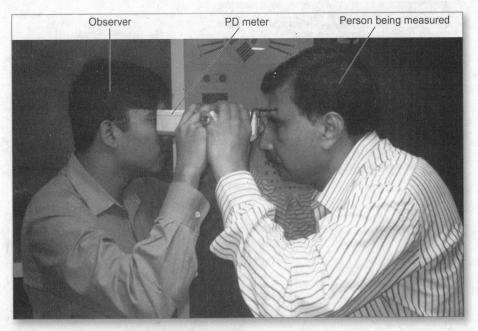

FIGURE 6.7: Dispenser and patient at same level

infinity for distance PD measurement using viewing distance adjustment lever.

3. Hold the pupillometer from the dispenser side and put the forehead rest against the forehead of the patient with rubber removable pads on nose. You may ask the client to hold the instrument for support.

4. Ask the patient to keep both eyes open.

5. For monocular distance PD use the eye occluding lever to occlude LE first to measure RE pupillary distance and then RE to measure the LE pupillary distance.

6. Ask the client to focus on the target light and move the left or right eye monocular PD adjustment lever, to align the centric line with the corneal reflex.

7. When measurement is over, all measurement would appear on the digital display. The result of monocular distance PD and total distance will automatically be recorded on the instrument.

OPTICIAN'S RULER

Using optician's ruler, IPD is measured with reference to any of the following three references:

1. From the geometrical center of the right pupil to the geometrical center of the left pupil.

2. From nasal limbus of RE to temporal limbus of LE.

3. From temporal limbus of RE to nasal limbus of LE

Measuring monocular distance PD using optician's ruler is done by following steps:

1. Patient and optician should place themselves directly opposite to each other at a distance of approximately 40 cm at the same eye level.

2. The optician places the ruler across the subject's nose with measuring edge tilted back so that it rests on the most recessed part of the nose as shown in Figure 6.8.

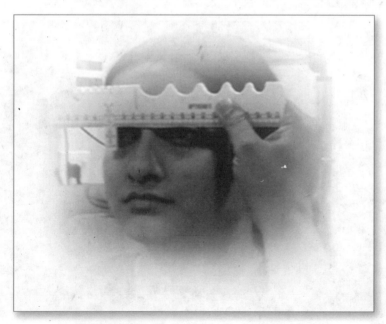

FIGURE 6.8: Placing optician's ruler to measure PD

3. The optician holds the PD ruler between thumb and forefinger and steadies his hand by placing his remaining three fingers against patient's head.

4. Occlude the patient's LE and ask the patient to focus his RE onto your LE and then lines up the 0 mark with the center of the pupil of patient's RE and note the scale reading of the ruler at the center of the nose as shown in Figure 6.9.

5. This gives you monocular distance PD for RE.

6. Now occlude his RE and ask him to look at your RE. Read the scale-reading where the RE center of pupil is lined up on the ruler as shown in Figure 6.10.

7. This gives you monocular distance PD for LE.

8. Make a record of the measured IPD.

Measuring monocular pupillary distance is very important when the eyes are asymmetrically placed, where the lens prescription is high, and where the two lens power has big difference.

Measuring binocular near PD using optician's ruler.

1. Patient and optician should place themselves directly opposite to each other at a distance of approximately 40 cm at the same eye level.

2. The optician places the ruler across the subject's nose with measuring edge tilted back so that it rests on the most recessed part of the nose.

3. The optician holds the PD rule between thumb and forefinger and steadies his hand by placing his remaining three fingers against patient's head.

4. Point the finger directly in line with the patient's nose and ask him to fixate at pointed finger with both eyes open as shown in Figure 6.11.

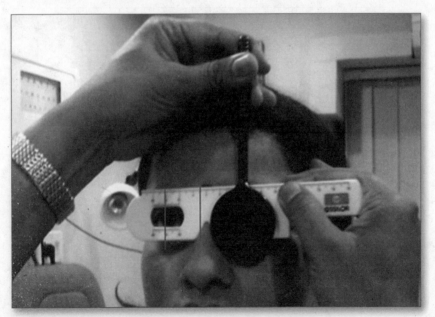

FIGURE 6.9: RE monocular distant IPD

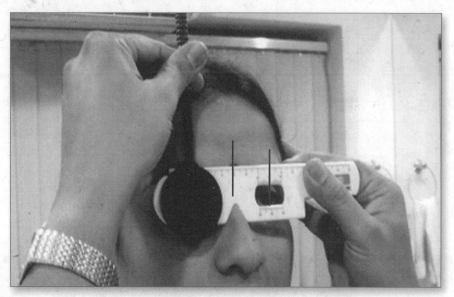

FIGURE 6.10: LE monocular distant IPD

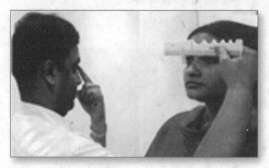

FIGURE 6.11: Asking the client to focus on pointed finger

5. Now line up the 0 mark with the center of the pupil of patient's RE as shown in Figure 6.12.
6. Note the scale reading of the ruler at the point where the LE center of pupil is being lined up as shown in Figure 6.13.
7. Now read the distance from 0 to the number where the LE center of pupil is being lined up.
8. The result so derived is the near PD in mm.

IPD measurement in some unusual situation like unequal pupil size and squint needs careful attention. In case of unequal pupil size, IPD should be measured with reference to the edges of the pupil. Two readings should be taken from both edges of the pupil and the actual measurement is the mean result of the two readings. Similarly when a patient has squint, measurement of IPD should be taken with reference to inner canthus of one eye to outer canthus of the other eye. The reading so taken will be good enough for normal purpose as small amount of prismatic effect will not be very important. Alternatively, one eye may be occluded and the optician ruler is centered on the unoccluded eye and then other eye is occluded and final reading is taken on the ruler over the unoccluded eye.

OPTICAL CENTER PLACEMENT

IPD is measured to place the optical center of the lens in the frame while edging and

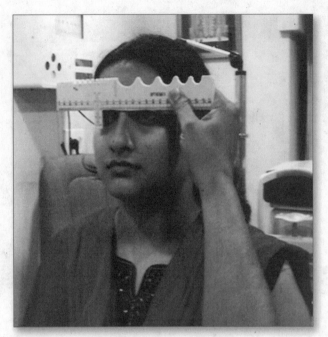

FIGURE 6.12: Aligning the 0 mark with RE center of pupil

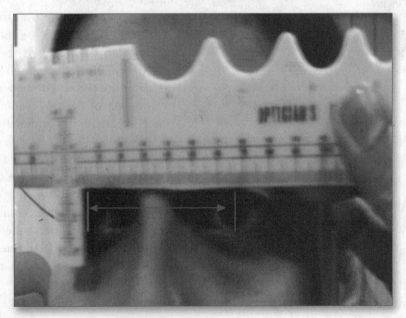

FIGURE 6.13: Near IPD

fitting the lens into the frame. Monocular values of IPD are considered to coincide with the optical center of each lens for distance vision and binocular near IPD is

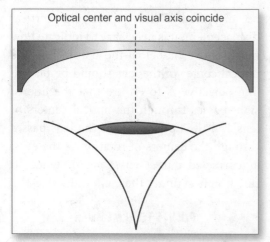

FIGURE 6.14: Optical center coincides with visual axis

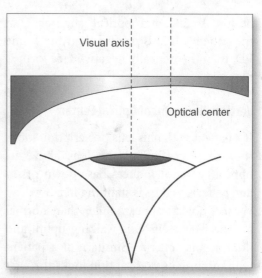

FIGURE 6.15: Decentration produces prismatic effect

considered to coincide with optical center of the lens for near vision. Both horizontal and vertical placement of optical centers are important for optical center placement to ensure that the visual axis passes through optical center of the lens as shown in Figure 6.14, and to prevent any prismatic effect through the lens that may be produced because of misalignment as shown in Figure 6.15.

Horizontal Placement of Optical Center

The optical centers of the lenses are placed at the same distance apart as the wearer's line of sight in order to prevent prismatic effect. At optical center of the lens there is no prismatic effect. The amount of induced prism depends on the power of the lens and the distance by which the optical center is displaced. It is calculated by Prentice's rule. When the prism is prescribed, optical center of the lens is not placed in front of the pupil center. Instead a point is found out where the amount of prism equals the prescribed prism. This new point on the lens is called

the major reference point (MRP) and is placed at patient's line of sight. So when prism is prescribed optical center and MRP may be at two different positions on the lens. While placing the optical center at desired IPD, following care should be taken:

1. If the wearer's eyes are at different distances from the nose, optical center must be placed with monocular PD.
2. If the two lenses are of two different powers, optical center must be placed with monocular PD.

There is also a relationship between the placement of optical center in the frame and the extent to which the "face form wrap" is applied. Face form wrap is a very important frame fitting criteria not only for cosmetic reasons but also for aligning the optical center of the lenses with the line of sight of each eye when directed straight forward. If the patient's PD is equal to the frame PD, then no face form is required, if the wearer's PD is less than the frame PD, positive face form wrap is required allowing both cosmetic and optical alignment. If the patient's IPD is greater than the frame PD, then theoretically negative face form is required.

Vertical Placement of Optical Center

If a patient with plus lens prescription looks through a portion of the lens above its optical center, it induces base down prism and he feels as if he is standing in a bowl, all vertical objects appears taller than normal and he feels as if he is walking uphill and floor seems concave. Similarly if a patient with minus lens prescription looks through a portion of the lens above its optical center, it induces base up prism and he feels as if he is standing on a hilltop, floor seems convex, vertical objects seem shorter than normal and he feels like a person who is walking downhill. This is the reason why vertical position of optical center is also very important. The optical center of the lens should be placed 3–4 mm below the pupil with the head erect for a frame with a pantoscopic tilt of 6°–8°. This is in line with the rule of thumb that says for every 2° pantoscopic tilt, the optical center should be lowered by 1 mm. If the lenses are only for near, the optical center may be placed slightly lower than the distance vision lenses. Spectacle frame are usually designed so that the pupil falls a few millimeter above the datum line, and this takes care of the difficulties automatically. But it is always wise to observe the frame fitting on the face and if needed the optical center should be displaced. While specifying vertical displacement, it is necessary to indicate how much above or below the datum line the optical center of the lens should be placed. The objective is to ensure that the line of sight passes through the optical centers of lens and the optical axis of the lens passes through the centers of rotation of the eyes, as corrected curve lenses are designed to function best under these circumstances.

POINTS TO REMEMBER

- The IPD is the distance from the center of one pupil to the center of the other pupil measured in millimeter.
- Monocular distance PD is taken by measuring the distance from the center of the pupil to the center of the nose.
- Failure to determine the IPD correctly results in a displacement of the optical center of the lens that requires the patient to turn his eyes inward or outward, patient keeps experiencing double vision and notices decreased ability of the eyes to work as a team in binocular vision.
- Where the eyes are asymmetrically placed, where the lens prescription is high, and where the two lens power has big difference, it is specially important to use monocular PD measurement.
- Essilor pupilometer measures the PD using a corneal reflex.
- When the prisms are prescribed optical center of the lens is not placed in front of the pupil center.
- The optical center of the lens should be placed 3–4 mm below the pupil with the head erect for a frame with a pantoscopic tilt of 6°–8°.

MULTIFOCAL SEGMENT HEIGHT MEASUREMENTS

Benjamin Franklin is credited with creating the first multifocal lenses. Prior to Franklin's invention, anyone with presbyopia had to carry two pairs of lenses—one for seeing distant objects and another for seeing up-close. There have been many changes to bifocal lenses since Franklin's original design, making these two-power lenses thinner, lighter and more attractive. Today, when you talk about multifocal lenses, there are different types of segmented and nonsegmented multifocal lenses. Dispensing multifocal lenses is one of the biggest challenges. The objective of Chapter 7 is to address the challenges associated with measuring vertical heights of segmented multifocal lenses.

Multifocal lenses are designed to provide vision at various distances from distance to near. They are available in segmented and nonsegmented lens design. The currently popular segmented type multifocal lens designs available are Univis D type, E-style and round segment bifocal lenses. Progressive addition lenses are most popular among the nonsegmented lens category which will be discussed in a separate chapter. In a multifocal lens optical correction for distance vision is provided at the top of the lens and optical correction for near vision is provided at the bottom of the lens. This is simply because distance objects are generally higher in the field of view and near objects are lower in the field of view, and an individual assumes a downward gaze angle of 25–30° to read at near viewing distance. The success depends a lot on correct placement of near segment of segmented multifocal lenses. Two measurements are very critical for placing the near segment of the segmented multifocal lenses:

1. Vertical position of near segment
2. Horizontal position of near segment.

VERTICAL POSITION OF NEAR SEGMENT

The vertical position of near segment is determined by the height of the top portion of the near segment that should not interfere with the distance vision in straight ahead gaze. Lower lid margin is usually taken as reference point for measuring the height of the segment. Some researchers advocate lower limbus as reference point for the purpose. However, the difference is mostly academic, since they are usually in approximately same position. If the lower lid is unusually lower than the lower limbus margin, the lower limbus margin makes a more consistent reference point. Segmezur, Seg Hi, Bernell segment gauge and optician's ruler are several tools that are used for segment height measurement. Among all optician ruler is the most commonly used tool for vertical height measurement of the near segment and the measurement is done using the actual frame on the wearer's eyes. The distance is measured with the scale extending downward and 0 point aligned with the lower lid margin or limbus to the lowest point where the lowest section of the inside edge of the lower eyewire intersects the scale, +0.5 mm to allow for the depth of the bevel. The lowest portion of the eyewire must be used, even if it is not precisely under the limbus. This can be best explained with the aviator shape frame as shown in Figure 7.1 in which case the distance from the top of the segment to the eyewire immediately below it is significantly different from the distance to the lowest point of the eyewire.

HORIZONTAL POSITION OF NEAR SEGMENT

Horizontal position of segment is specified as segment inset. Segment inset is specified as the difference between the patient's distance PD and near PD. In the normal range of PDs, the near PD for a reading distance of 40 cm is 4 mm less than the distance PD. Segment inset, therefore, is usually specified as 2 mm for each lens. There are two reasons for insetting bifocal segment—to ensure that the patient's line of sight passes through the segment at its optical center and to ensure that the reading fields for the two segments will coincide with one another. The horizontal placement of near segment of Univis D bifocal is done with reference to near IPD during lens edging. However, for round shaped bifocal lenses, there is a need for making provision for segment inset while lens surfacing in case of cylinder lens power. This is achieved by altering the cylinder axis during lens surfacing. A change in axis by 5° rotates the near segment in by 1 mm. The required cylinder axis in right eye is subtracted from the given cylinder axis and

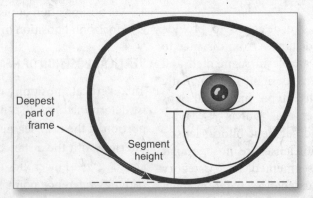

FIGURE 7.1: Measuring the segment height from the lowest portion of the eyewire

an equal degree of rotation is added to the given left eye cylinder axis. For example, we need to move the near segment in by 2 mm for the following lens prescription:

- RE –1.00 Dsph/ –1.00 Dcyl @180°
- LE –1.00 Dsph/ –1.00 Dcyl @180°
- BE Near Add + 2.00 Dsph

In this case in order to make provision for 2 mm segment inset in right eye, given cylinder axis will be altered by 10°. Therefore, while lens surfacing the lens power will be altered for the purpose of surfacing as under:

- RE –1.00 Dsph/ –1.00 Dcyl @170°
- LE –1.00 Dsph/ –1.00 Dcyl @10°
- BE Near Add + 2.00 Dsph

However, lenses will be edged and fitted at 180° only.

SEQUENTIAL STEPS TO MEASURE THE SEGMENT HEIGHT

The most accurate and consistent measurement of segment height can be taken by using optician ruler. The segment height can be mentioned either with reference to the datum line or with reference to the lower eyewire and is given as the top end of the near segment, say 20 mm, above lower eyewire or 2 mm below the datum line. A typical routine procedure for taking the measurement is:

1. Adjust the selected frame for necessary pantoscopic tilt, face form wrap and nose pads fitting as shown in Figure. 7.2.
   - 6°–8° of pantoscopic tilt is considered to be cosmetically acceptable.
   - Adjust the frame for positive face form wrap.
   - In case of metal frames adjust the nose pads for frontal, splay and vertical angle.
2. Ask the patient to stand or sit at your eye level. Put the adjusted frame on the patient's face and ask him to look straight ahead at your eyes. It is suggested that the positions of the segment top should be measured when the head is held straight ahead and the viewing gaze of the patient is in primary gaze position. Put the frame on the patient's face and direct him to look straight into your eyes. If necessary, adjust the height of your chair so that your eyes are on the same level as patients (Fig. 7.3).
3. If the frame is without demonstration lens, attach a vertical strip of transparent adhesive tape to each eye of the frame as

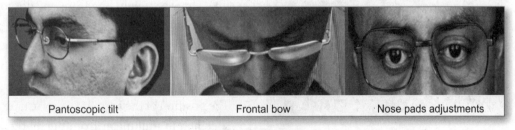

| Pantoscopic tilt | Frontal bow | Nose pads adjustments |

FIGURE 7.2: Frame fitting

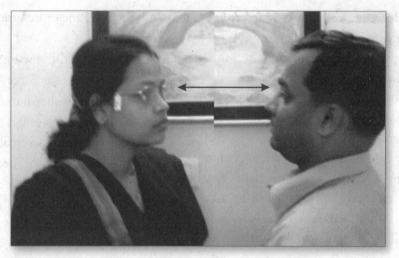

FIGURE 7.3: Position of the patient and optician

shown in Figure 7.4 to enable reference points to be marked.

4. Direct the patient to look straight into your open left eyes and using a fine tip marking pen, place dots at the same height as the lower edge of the patient's right lower eyelid. Similarly, without moving his head, also mark in front of the patient's left lower lid as shown in Figure 7.5.

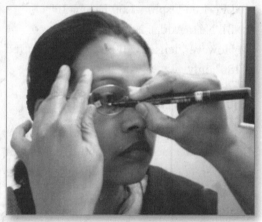

FIGURE 7.5: Marking on lens insert with reference to lower lid

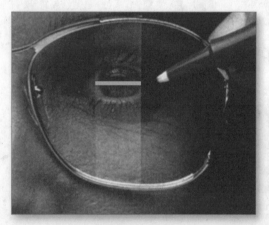

FIGURE 7.4: Tap on frame eyewire

5. Remove the frame and put the frame face down with dots coinciding with a straight line. Draw a straight line from one dot to another as shown in Figure 7.6.

6. Put back the frame on the face and verify. The marked line should be in line with lower eye lid as shown in Figure 7.7.

7. The position of the segment top is usually specified in millimeter from the marked

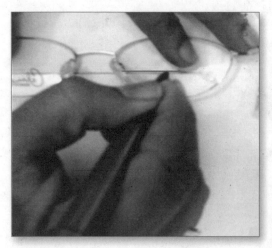

FIGURE 7.6: Marking straight line on lens insert

straight line to the lower eyewire of the frame where the bevel of the lens will fit into the groove which can be measured with ruler as shown in Figure 7.8.

VERIFYING THE POSITION OF SEGMENT HEIGHT

The measured segment height can be verified for its accuracy by the subjective response of the patient very effectively. The patient is asked to stand and look straight ahead. A card is held over the lower half of the frame with its upper border coinciding with the proposed segment position as shown in Figure 7.9. The patient should be able to see the floor over the top of the card at a distance of 15 feet.

Now ask the subject to look down at the reading material. The card is held over the upper portion of the frame with its lower border at the level of the proposed bifocal segment. The reading material should be visible without major readjustments of the subject's posture or reading material.

DISPENSING SEGMENTED MULTIFOCAL LENSES

Several factors determine the vertical position of the near segment of multifocal lenses. In all normal cases the top end of near segment is placed in line with lower eyelid of the patient. However, certain occupational needs, unusual reading posture, patient's height and past habits also influence the position. If a person who habitually holds

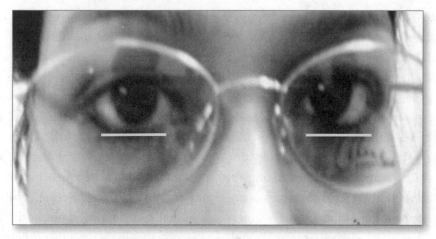

FIGURE 7.7: Marked line is in line with lower eyelid

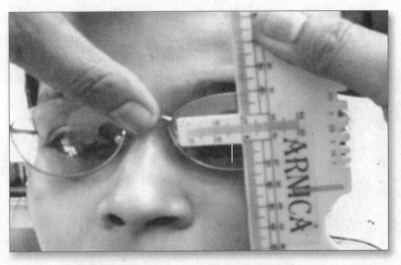

FIGURE 7.8: Measuring vertical height of near segment

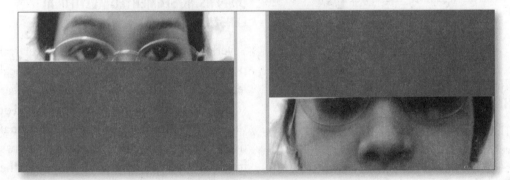

FIGURE 7.9: Verifying for segment height

his head high will need a lower segment height than a person who slouches a bit and keeps his head downward. A tall person who habitually keeps his head down may need a little higher segment top whereas a short height person who has to keep his head up may prefer a little down segment top. Past wearing habit of the subject should also be given importance while positioning the segment top. If a wearer is used to wearing bifocal segment up, fitting a lower segment in the new spectacle will create trouble for him to adjust immediately. A patient who works more at the desk will prefer an unusually high segment and will learn to keep head down for certain distance work. If the patient's lower lid is unusually lower, with sclera showing underneath limbus, he may be more comfortable if the measurement is taken from lower limbus. The vertical position of bifocal segment height is very important because a lower height may lead a patient complaining about neck stiffness, whereas the higher segment height may create obstruction during distance viewing gaze. When one eye is higher than the other, a difference in prescribed segment heights may be required so that the person's eyes meet the bifocal line simultaneously on down gaze. Vertex distance of the lens also influences the vertical position of the segment top as a bifocal lens that is farther away from the eyes will interfere with the vision just as if they were placed higher. In case vertical prisms are prescribed with a bifocal lens, the segment height should be displaced from its original location in the direction of apex by 0.3 mm for every diopter of prism. The near segment shape also influences the vertical position of near segment.

Invisible Seamless Bifocal Lenses

Invisible bifocals are one-piece bifocal lenses having round segment, in which the line of demarcation between the distance portion of the lens and the bifocal segment

has been obliterated. Optically the lens performs the same as a standard round shaped bifocal, as only two actual zones of focus exist—one for distance and the other for near. The obliteration process produces distortion around the bifocal segment which varies in width from less than 3 mm to just under 5 mm, depending on the power of the near addition and the base curve. This area serves as the boundary of the segment and permits the lens to be fitted according to the same provisions that affect an ordinary round bifocal. Since the blending is wider than the actual demarcation line, the bifocal may require either slightly higher placement of the top of the segment or greater depression of the gaze for reading. The manufacturer recommends fitting this bifocal little higher than other types of bifocal lenses. Approximately 2 mm above round shape bifocal is most commonly practiced as shown in Figure 7.10.

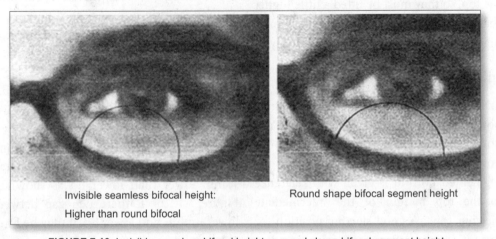

Invisible seamless bifocal height: Higher than round bifocal

Round shape bifocal segment height

FIGURE 7.10: Invisible seamless bifocal height vs round shape bifocal segment height

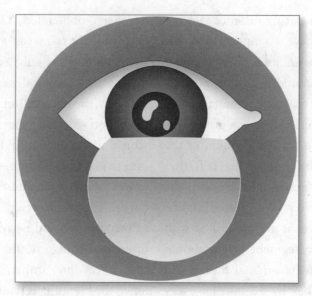

FIGURE 7.11: Trifocal segment height position

Round Shape Bifocal Lenses

Round segment bifocal have a segment with a dividing line that is a single circular arc which is least visible compared to the other bifocals. When placed at the bottom half of the lens, they are often called 'Down Curve' bifocal lenses. The centre of the segment in round shape bifocal falls much below from the top, so they must be fitted a little higher than the other bifocals. Approximately 1 mm higher than D Bifocal works wonderfully.

Trifocal

Trifocal is characterized by three separate portions of different powers—distance portion, near portion and intermediate portion. The ideal position for placing the segmented portion is given with reference to the top margin of the intermediate viewing zone. A good starting position for the Intermediate Portion top is at or just below the lower pupil margin as shown in Figure 7.11.

E-style Bifocal

E-style bifocal is one piece bifocal lens with two different curves ground usually on the front surface. The optical center of both the distance and the near lens lies on the dividing line. It is, therefore, classified as monocentric bifocal. The difference in curves between the distance and the near portion of the lens produces a ledge that is most prominent towards the outer edge of the lens. The optical center of the distance and near portion lies on the dividing line that minimize vertical image jump. Also because of distinctive dividing line, it should ideally be fitted approximately 1 mm lower than lower lid as shown in Figure 7.12 or if there is a gap between lower limbus and lower lid, it may be fitted at lower lid height.

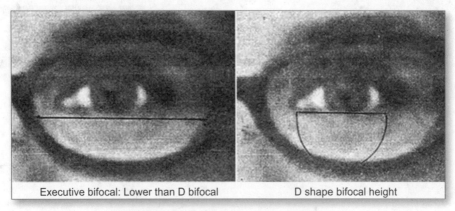

| Executive bifocal: Lower than D bifocal | D shape bifocal height |

FIGURE 7.12: Trifocal segment height position

POINTS TO REMEMBER

- The lower lid margin is most commonly used as a reference point for measuring bifocal segment height.
- The measurements for segment heights should be done using only the actual frame that will be worn.
- The bifocal segment height is measured with reference to the position of the lower lid to the point where the lowest section of the inside edge of the lower eyewire intersects the scale, plus 0.5 mm to allow for depth of the bevel.
- The total bifocal segment inset is the difference between the distance PD and near PD of a patient.
- A crooked frame will result in unequal segment height measurements.
- A person who is accustomed to an unusually high segment position should again be fitted with same bifocal segment height.
- If the segment height of a bifocal lens is too low, the wearer will complain of neck stiffness.
- When one eye is higher than the other, a difference in prescribed segment heights may be required so that the person's eyes will meet the bifocal line simultaneously on down gaze.
- If the bifocal lenses are farther from the eye, they interfere with the vision just as if they were placed higher.
- For every diopter of vertical prism, the segment height should be displaced from its original location in the direction of apex by 0.3 mm.

DISPENSING IN MYOPIA

Myopia or nearsightedness is a condition wherein the patient has more difficulty seeing distant objects than the near objects. There are different types of surgical and nonsurgical correction modalities that are available to correct myopia. Spectacle dispensing is one of the most common nonsurgical modalities and dispensing spectacle poses lots of challenges. Chapter 8 talks about these challenges and explains the ways to address these challenges.

Myopia is a form of refractive error where light rays from infinity falls in front of the retina when the eye is at rest. Mostly myopia is because of the increased corneal or lens surface curvature, a shallow anterior chamber, higher refractivity of the crystalline lens or larger axial length of the globe. A myope cannot see at long distance, but he can see at closer distance. The visual acuity is seriously affected that interferes with daily activities. Accommodation is of no value to myope, in fact it increases the difficulties of the myopes. The patient has no means to overcome his deficiency other than correcting for the error. Myopia can develop at any age. However it has a tendency to develop in childhood or teenage and it gets worse as you get older before it stables at around adulthood. Sometimes there may be episodes where myopia continues to increase even after adulthood. High myopia is usually because your eye has grown in length. This means that even though your eyes are healthy, you are at a higher risk of developing eye conditions and changes associated with the lengthening of the eye. Myopia can be classified as:

- Low myopia ranging between –0.25 D to –3.00 D.
- Moderate myopia ranging between –3.00 D to –6.00 D.
- High myopia ranging anywhere above –6.00 D.

The nonsurgical treatment of myopia is the correction of error either by spectacle lenses or contact lenses. In low myopia full correction restores the vision and not much interference is needed on a regular basis. Usually in low myopia change in refractive error is not seen after the age of adolescence. In high myopia, the full correction can rarely be tolerated. An attempt is made to undercorrect as little as is compatible with comfort for binocular near vision. Usually an undercorrection to the tune of 1.00D to 3.00 D or even more may be required, depending upon the age of the patient and degree of myopia. Undercorrection is always better to avoid near vision problem and minifications of images.

Most patients are looking for thinner and lighter lens that hides the lens power and makes the spectacles cosmetically appealing on their face. The dispensing optician follows the general principle of smaller size for high minus prescription to provide thinner and lighter spectacle. However, lens thickness can be reduced not only by smaller frame size, but also by judicious selection of the frame shape and appropriate higher refractive index of the lens material. A symmetrical shape of the spectacle frame enhances the overall appeal of the lenses. High refractive index lens material can reduce lens thickness which can also be designed in aspherical lens design to provide flatter look to the lens. Thus lens material selection is critical for myopes and lens designs can be appropriately selected to enhance the overall visual performance and cosmetic value. The challenges associated

with optical dispensing in case of moderate to high myopia are shown in Flowchart 8.1.

MINIMIZING LENS THICKNESS

The edge thickness of the minus lenses is the first concern of all myopic patients. Minimizing edge thickness of the minus lens is a real challenge for the dispensing opticians. The following guidelines help:

1. Smaller frame size always helps minimizing the edge thickness of the minus lenses and allows a thinner edge profile of the lenses. However, while selecting the appropriate size for a patient; make sure that the temple width of the frame encompasses the facial width of the wearer.

   Symmetrical shapes with least frame difference are most ideal for uniform thickness from all around. Square, round shape or broader oval shape frames are good to ensure uniform thickness from all around in high minus prescription. Steep rectangular shape creates a disparity in lens edge thickness between temporal and nasal side of the frame.

2. Several mid and high-index lens materials are available; they allow thinner lens profile in moderate to high myopia because of increased light bending

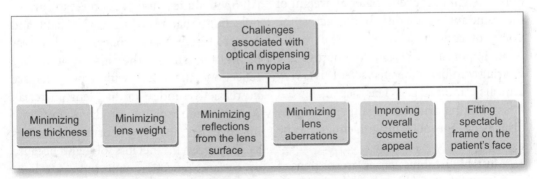

FLOWCHART 8.1: Challenges associated with optical dispensing in myopia

ability of the lens material. However, two more factors should be considered while selecting the appropriate refractive index of the lens material—they are Abbe value and density of the lens material.

3. Use of aspheric lens design provides flatter lens form that improves the lens cosmetic value.

4. Use of edge treatments and modifications as to the bevel design may also help to minimize the apparent thickness of the lenses. Polishing the bevel is one of the simplest ways in case of plastic lens material. Avoiding conventional V-bevel design also helps; the mini-bevel technique can provide effective results.

5. Lens edge thickness may be distributed uniformly between front and the back portion of the eyewire; they also effectively minimize the apparent lens thickness.

6. Decentration of optical center is also effective to ensure the uniform lens thickness at both nasal and temporal portion of the frame by fitting the lens with reference to geometrical center of the lens rather than optical center.

MINIMIZING LENS WEIGHT

The overall weight of the spectacle comprises of the weight of the lens material, weight of the frame and weight distribution across the points of contact. Minimizing the weight is an important criterion to improve the wearing comfort of the spectacle. This is very critical for mineral glass lens dispensing, but it is not as important in organic plastic lens dispensing. The following guidelines may be useful:

1. Most high minus lenses are dispensed with high-index lens material. High-index lens materials have higher density that leads to increase in lens material weight. Therefore, care should be taken to select the appropriate index of the lens material for the given lens prescription. It is prudent to compare the percentage reduction in lens thickness against the percentage gain in lens material weight while selecting the appropriate refractive index of the material.

2. The weight of the lens can also be minimized by working with the smaller size of the spectacle frame. Smaller size reduces lens mass and thereby minimizes the lens weight. The overall weight of the spectacle depends upon the weight of the frames, lens size, lens mass and also on lens material.

3. The weight of the spectacle as a whole is usually borne entirely by the bearing surface of the frame on bridge of the nose. Larger the bearing surface, more evenly the weight of the frame is spread around the contact area. This is possible only in case of plastic frame. Glass lenses fitted with smaller nose pads of metal frames are the worst possible scenario.

MINIMIZING REFLECTIONS FROM THE LENS SURFACE

All ophthalmic lenses are subject to surface reflections that result in loss of light and compromised visual appeal of the eyes behind the lenses. The amount of surface reflection increases with the increase in refractive index of the lens material. Antireflection coating produces dramatic improvement in the performance of lens as they prevent the loss of light because of surface reflection and increases light transmission. They also add to the cosmetic appeal of the lens by reducing the intensity of reflections to the point that they are almost invisible. Some efforts may also be made to minimize the effect of surface reflection by altering the pantoscopic tilt, changing the vertex distance, selecting the smaller size and with patient education and counseling. The lens edging leaves a fine-ground edge that acts as diffusely reflecting surface. The reflection of edges at the back surface can be seen through the front surface as myopic concentric rings (Fig. 8.1). This is very annoying to the wearer. In organic plastic lenses it is easier to polish the edge and fit into the frame, but polishing is difficult in case of glass lens material. Rubbing the lens edges with graphite pencil all over or apply any concentrated oil before mounting the lenses into the frame is a simple technique that ages the lens and minimizes the appearance of concentric rings.

MINIMIZING LENS ABERRATIONS

The on-axis or central portion performance of the lens provides perfect vision. But the off-axis lens portion degrades and deforms the image quality and thus limits the field of clear vision through the lenses. In other words, rays of light behaves best when they pass through the optical center of the lens, i.e. when the rays of light pass through the optical axis of the lens, but as the wearer's line of sight makes an angle to the optical axis of the lens, incident rays of light are no longer brought to a single-point focus at the desired focal point of the lens. There is an error in focus which is known as lens aberration. The effect of lens aberration increases with the larger angle that the line of sight makes with the optical axis. This effect is more noticed with higher lens power. The following guidelines may be useful to minimize the effect of lens aberration:

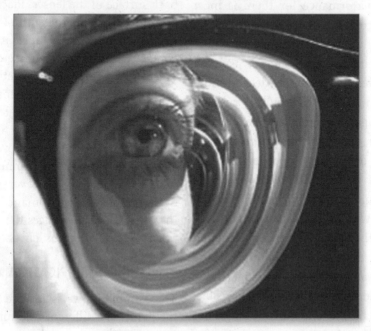

FIGURE 8.1: Concentric myopic ring

1. Correct base curve is selected in order to ensure that the wearer enjoys a wider field of clear vision.
2. A judicious selection of lens material is being done with higher Abbe value.
3. Aspheric lens surface is chosen to minimize the effect of oblique astigmatism by creating surface astigmatism.
4. The lens should be fitted as close to the eyes as permitted by eyelashes. A close fitting has an advantage of improved retinal image quality.

IMPROVING OVERALL COSMETIC APPEAL

High myopes are usually most sensitive to the cosmetic value of their spectacle. They are most conscious about the lens edge thickness. Typically the first thing they observe in their spectacle is the lens thickness and the myopic concentric rings. The visual performance for them is most often the secondary. Therefore, all factors like smaller frame size, symmetrical frame shape, high-index lens material, aspheric lens design, bevel placement, decentration, antireflection coating, edge polish, rubbing the lens edges by graphite pencil and dark thicker rimmed frames are critical. A judicious decision is to be made as to apply one or more of the techniques. The amount of minification may be minimized by working with vertex distances and lens curvature. The use of antireflective coating makes eyes more visible, eliminates the "glassy" appearance of mid- and high-index materials, and it makes the lenses less visible. It can almost be like removing the lenses but leaving the prescription in place.

FITTING SPECTACLE FRAME ON THE PATIENT'S FACE

Thicker and heavier minus lenses creates certain mechanical issues that hinders appropriate placement of the spectacle frame on the patient's face. Spectacles are fitted so that there is a comfortable distance from the eye to the back surface of the lenses such that the eye lashes do not make contact with it. There are so many predisposing factors that include unusually long lashes, frame wrap, facial anatomy, lens form, position of the lens bevel and lens prescription. Positive face form wrap brings the back surface of the lens closer to the eyelashes and thus increases the probability of lashes brushing against the back surface of the lenses. Steeper curve prevents eyelashes brushing against the lens back surface. While mounting the lenses into the frame the placement of bevel also helps preventing contact of lashes with back surface of the lenses. Placing the bevel at front edge shifts the entire lens thickness inside which increases the possibility of lash contact with the back surface of the lenses. This also hinders nose pads adjustments in case of metal frame. Placement of the bevel at center divides the overall lens thickness equally visible from outside and inside. It not only increases the vertex distance but also makes the lens look thinner apparently. Vertex distance is also very critical for optimum visual performance as increase in vertex distance reduces the effective lens power in case of minus lenses.

DISPENSING IN MYOPIC ASTIGMATISM

The astigmatic eye is unique in the sense that it has two different amount of refractive error in each of the two principal meridians.

Patients with astigmatism cannot achieve clarity of vision by holding an object at any single position. This is unlike a myope, who can bring the object closer and read clearly; neither will accommodative effort help the astigmatic patient achieve proper focus as it does for the pre-presbyopic hyperope. The only remedy for the patients with astigmatism, is optical correction. Myopic astigmatism is corrected by minus cylinder lenses. Cylinder lenses have different power in its two principle meridians. The power along the axis meridian results from the sphere alone, whereas the power at right angles to the axis meridian is the sum of the spherical and the cylinder. The lenses create line images instead of point image, the orientation of which depends upon the axis of the cylinder lens. In simple myopic astigmatism eye, one meridian is plain and the other has minus correction. In compound myopic astigmatism, both the meridians have corrections, but they differ in magnitude. Thus for a prescription -5.00 Dsph / -1.00 Dcyl at $90°$, the power along the $90°$ is -5.00 D and the power along $180°$ is -6.00 D. The resultant edge thickness at $90°$ would be less than that of at $180°$. Whenever possible, the lens shape chosen for an astigmatic prescription should have its maximum diameter coincident with the minimum power meridian of the lens. The straight forward meaning is that the position of maximum edge thickness varies with the cylinder axis direction.

Astigmatic lenses for myopia provides the best optical performance when the cylinder is incorporated on the back surface of the lens—the lenses are supplied as minus-base toric design. Minus-base toric construction also improves the appearance of the lens, since the variation in edge thickness that occurs along the different power meridian can be hidden on the back of the lens. However, for a deep minus lens, it is easier for the manufacturer to incorporate the cylinder on the front surface of the lens in the form of plano-convex cylinder surface.

Nonuniform image minification by a sphero-cylinder lens sometimes causes meridional aniseikonia which produces disturbances in spatial orientation. A common complaint is that flat surfaces appear tilted. However, almost always, the patient will rapidly adapt to these initial symptoms, which cease to be annoying. A strange distortion in which case square or rectangular objects looked trapezoidal is very common, specially when the astigmatic prescription is stronger than necessary or axis is incorrect. The difficulties can be simply alleviated by reducing the amount of astigmatic correction, while maintaining the spherical equivalent.

Another important issue is the correct shape of the frame while dispensing high astigmatic lenses. Shapes like round and oval shape which do not have any sharp corners should be avoided as there is a possibility of disorientation of axis.

FACTORS THAT INFLUENCE ADAPTATION

Patients with high myopia are self-motivated as they know that they are handicapped without their spectacle or lenses and they need to use their spectacle to perform their everyday task. The first thing they look for in the morning is their own spectacle. They do not readily accept changes. Base curve of the lens, face form wrap of the frame, pantoscopic angle of the frame, vertex distance—all influence the adaptation with lenses. They develop adaptation to a particular lens form and are often dissatisfied when their lens form is changed. Some sensitive patients do not accept the change in refractive index of the lens material. Since myopic patients are more centrally aware they readily notice any defects in lenses that may also create adaptation issue if not resolved. Changing from flatter lens form to steeper lens form or vice versa, increasing the front wrap angle of frame front, increasing the frame size and the vertex distance of the frame and altering the cylinder side—all can have negative impact on adaption.

Minus spectacle lenses have the effect of base-out prisms. It means the patient needs to accommodate to read. Accommodation induces secondarily convergence. The patient needs to converge for binocular fixation at near, with minus correction. Reducing minus correction, therefore, may alter accommodative and convergence mechanism that may produce symptomatic effect. Besides, image minifications and barrel type distortions are other, noticed distortion with high minus lenses to which the patient adapts. Any change in minus prescription may bring in unpleasant optical effects to which the patient may object. Minus lenses decreases light scatter and increases light intensity, the effect is noticed as increases in contrast. When the minus power is reduced the patient may feel reduced visual performance through the lens for initial few days.

POINTS TO REMEMBER

- Myopia is a condition in which rays of light coming from infinity focus before retina.
- Change in vertex distance significantly influences the effective power of the lens.
- Myopes are often accustomed to a particular lens form and often dissatisfied when their lens form is changed.
- Placing the bevel at the front edge shifts the entire lens thickness inside, that hinders nose pad adjustments in high minus lens prescription.
- Astigmatic cylinder for myopes provides best optical performance when the cylinder is incorporated on the back surface as minus cylinder.

DISPENSING IN HYPERMETROPIA

Hypermetropia or farsightedness is a condition wherein the patient has more difficulty seeing near objects than the distant objects. The condition poses different challenges while dispensing lenses, some of them are absolutely unique to the condition. Chapter 9 talks about these challenges and explains the ways to address these challenges.

Hypermetropia is a refractive error in which parallel rays of light entering the eye reach a focal point behind the plane of the retina, while accommodation is maintained in a state of relaxation. In a hypermetropic eye the focal point is located behind the retina which may be brought to the retina by accommodation and therefore the patient can see the distant objects clearly by exerting accommodation. In the process he exerts all his accommodative ability to look at distant objects and cannot accommodate to look at near objects. Thus, he finds difficulty seeing near objects. Hypermetropia is of 3 types:

- Latent hypermetropia
- Manifest hypermetropia
- Absolute hypermetropia.

Latent hypermetropia can be totally by eye's own accommodative ability. It can be detected only by cycloplegia. Manifest hypermetropia can be corrected either by patient's own accommodation or by plus lens. Total hypermetropia is the sum of manifest and latent hypermetropia. Correction of hypermetropia depends upon patient's ability to compensate for close work and symptoms. In case of young patients, if it is not associated with accommodative strabismus, it may be avoided and in case of old patient, hypermetropia is corrected to improve near vision.

Plus lenses or convex lenses are used to correct hypermetropia. The cross-section shape of plus lens is different from the cross-section shape of minus lens. The mechanical problems encountered with plus lenses are therefore, different from that of the minus lenses. Therefore, dispensing in hypermetropia encounters different challenges; common among them are shown in Flowchart 9.1.

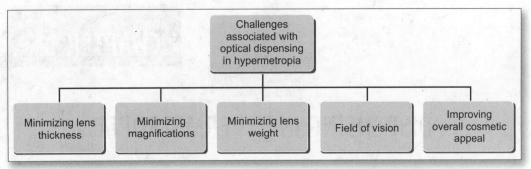

FLOWCHART 9.1: Challenges associated with optical dispensing in hypermetropia

MINIMIZING LENS THICKNESS

The edge of the minus lens reduces as it is edged down to fit the frame. A reasonably good finish can be obtained from the stock lenses. This is not possible with plus lenses. The edge thickness of plus lenses increases as the diameter is reduced. The only way of reducing edge thickness for finished diameter is surface the lens with full information as to prescription, decentration and frame size. The center thickness of the plus lens can be reduced by choosing a high refractive index material. Aspherical lens design can also be made with high refractive index material to flatten the lens surface and thereby reducing the sagittal height to minimize the apparent lens thickness.

MINIMIZING MAGNIFICATION

Each diopter of plus power leads to about 3% magnification of image. When the objects appear larger they appear falsely closer than reality, and this leads to physical incoordination. Magnification effect of the lens detracts from the overall appearance of the wearer, as the eyes and its surroundings appear more prominent since they are enlarged. This is a great challenge that can be addressed by:

1. Keeping the vertex distance of the lens as closer to eyes as permitted by eyelashes.
2. Use of flatter aspheric form lenses.

MINIMIZING LENS WEIGHT

The overall weight of the spectacle comprises of the weight of the lens material, weight of the frame and weight distribution across the points of contact. Minimizing the weight is an important criterion to improve the wearing comfort of the spectacle. This is very critical for mineral glass lens dispensing, but it is not as important in organic plastic lens dispensing. The following guidelines may be useful:

1. Most high plus lenses are dispensed with high-index lens material to reduce center thickness of the lens.
2. The weight of the lens can also be minimized by:
   - Smaller size of the spectacle frame, smaller size reduces lens mass and thereby minimizes the lens weight.
   - Lenses must be surfaced to the size of the frame.
   - Dispensing plastic frame where the entire weight of the spectacle is distributed on the larger bearing surface on bridge of the nose.

- Glass lenses fitted with smaller nose pads of metal frames are the worst possible scenario.
3. Lenticular lens design in organic plastic lens material is very good option for high plus lenses to reduce lens mass and edge thickness.

FIELD OF VISION

The higher magnifications produced by high plus lenses reduces the field of view through the high plus lenses. It produces a blind area or scotoma in the patient's periphery. It means the object disappears in between the field of view through the lens and the object field immediately visible outside the lens edge where the object reappears again. The presence of above scotoma leads to another unique phenomenon called "Jack-in-the-box". The object lying in the periphery of the patient's visual field is not clear as the light arising from the objects lying immediately near the lens edge does not pass through the lens as shown in Figure 9.1A. The patient only perceives the presence of object. The patient tends to move his head towards the object to see it clearly; the object comes to the area of scotoma and thus disappears as shown in Figure 9.1B. The patient turns his head further so that the object comes in front of the spectacle lenses in the visible area and thus it reappears as shown in Figure 9.1C. This sudden disappearance and reappearance of the objects is called Jack-in-the-box phenomenon.

The edge of a convex lens acts as a prism. The higher the power of the convex lens the greater is the prism angle. The light falling on the prism bends towards its base; therefore, greater the angle more will be the bending. In aphakic lenses, the light falling at the edge of the lens bends towards the center of the lens and does not reach the pupil and therefore they are not seen, resulting in a scotomatic area in the visual field. Since the edge of the lens is present all around the lens, it gives rise to a ring-shaped scotoma. The position of ring scotoma moves with the movement of eyes. It is, therefore, called "roving ring scotoma".

IMPROVING OVERALL COSMETIC APPEAL

There are two big challenges that are important for hypermetropic dispensing in order to improve the cosmetic appeal of the overall spectacle. They minimize the lens magnifications and the lens bulge. An

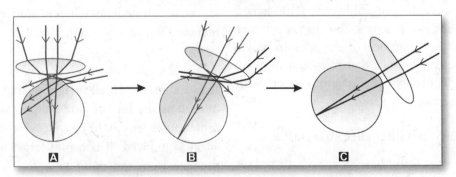

FIGURE 9.1: Restricted field of vision through high plus lens

enormous improvement is possible with the use of flatter aspheric lens forms. This is because in case of aspheric lenses not only the plate height of the lens is smaller but they also lie closer to the eyes, which makes them appear less bulbous. This implies that the appearance of patient's eyes and surrounding portions of the face are seen with less magnification than steeply curved spherical lens surface.

DISPENSING IN HYPERMETROPIC ASTIGMATISM

In simple hyperopic astigmatism, one image plane is located at retina, and the other is located behind the retina, whereas in compound hyperopic astigmatism, both the image planes are located at different distances behind the retina. Astigmatic lenses for plus lenses provides the best optical performance, when the cylinder is incorporated on the convex surface, the lenses being supplied as plus toric lenses. Plus base toric lenses, however, requires the lens laboratory to keep large range of toric tools. Hence most lens laboratories, given the choice incorporate the cylinder on the concave side as minus base toric. In high astigmatism this improves the cosmetic appearance of the spectacle, since the variation in lens edge thickness is hidden on the back of the lenses. But minus cylinder at the back surface of the lens increases the vertex distance that may lead to affect the effective lens power and interfere with vision quality.

FACTORS THAT INFLUENCE ADAPTATION

Plus lens creates base in effect and relaxes accommodation, and thereby minimizes the effort to converge. When the accommodation is deficient, plus lens aids accommodation. When a patient wears the plus correction there is a change in the accommodation and convergence mechanism of his visual system. He needs to establish a new relationship between accommodation and convergence mechanism of the visual system.

Each diopter of plus lens brings in 3% of magnification of the object, means the appeared object size is larger than what it is. The brain takes some time to adapt to this. The effect of magnification can be minimized by efficiently controlling the vertex distance and lens form. However, when the lens form is changed to aspherical from spherical, sometimes it bothers the hyperope as he misses the magnification.

The effect of plus lens is noticed as light scattering and thus reducing the light intensity. The person notices the effect as reduction in contrast. High plus lens also produces pincushion distortion to which brain adapts in course of use.

A patient with latent hypermetropia when corrected for it may also report blurriness of distance vision and good vision for near. Immediate relief is noticed by reducing the plus correction or the patient adapts to it in course of use.

Basic optics of the lens causes poor stabilization of retinal images during head motion as the line of gaze shifts from the center of the lens to the periphery, prismatic effect is induced. It becomes larger as the distance from the point to optical center increases.

POINTS TO REMEMBER

- The edge thickness of plus lens increases as the diameter is reduced.
- Each diopter of plus lens leads to a magnification of about 3% of image. Closer vertex distance minimizes the magnification effect.
- Flatter aspheric lens forms makes the lens appear less bulbous and also lies closer to the eyes reduces magnification effect.
- The sudden disappearance and reappearance of the objects in the field of view with plus lenses is called Jack-in-the-box phenomenon.
- Plus lens creates base in effect and relaxes accommodation, and thereby minimizes the effort to converge.

CHAPTER 10

DISPENSING IN PRESBYOPIA

Dispensing in presbyopia is not only a challenge but also an opportunity. Presbyopia occurs because the patient finds a reduction in his amplitude of accommodation. The range of clear vision is inadequate for the patient's commonly performed near and extended-near vision tasks. The difficulties are more in near distance than the intermediate distances. The bottom line is presbyopia is not just the problem of near vision at 40 cm, it is a problem of reduced vision at various reading distances. The patient who is working on computer also notices blur vision at the computer monitor which is usually kept at 50–70 cm. The blurring at this distance is comparatively less as accommodative demand at this distance is comparatively less. Those who are involved more in near vision tasks are likely to have more difficulty. Because the need to read and work at near and intermediate distances is important in all industrialized societies, presbyopia has both clinical and social significance. Chapter 10 highlights on these issues and acquaint the readers as to various correction options available in the form of various lens types and challenges associated with dispensing those lenses.

Presbyopia is an aging phenomenon that results in lot of changes in human ocular system. Most of the anatomical and physiological processes follow a gradual decline with the increasing age. The quality of vision worsens. Most important functional changes are noted in reduction in pupil size and the loss of accommodation or focusing capability. There is a substantial decrease in light received at the retina as compare to younger people and the individual starts complaining of difficulties in reading and other close works. The reasons are attributed to the gradual loss of lens capsule elasticity and a weakening of the ciliary muscle. Presbyopia is corrected with the additional plus correction and the amount of additional plus lens depends upon host factors:

1. Age.
2. Amplitude of accommodation.
3. Distance correction.
4. Occupations.
5. Reading habits, hobbies and other near vision demands.

6. Reading stature (long arms help delay the need for correction).

There is no evidence that the use of reading glasses retards or accelerates the further progression of presbyopia.

LENS OPTIONS

Presbyopia is a relative entity, and a number of conflicting requirements must be met and solved simultaneously before selecting a suitable lens type. A variety of lens types are available for optical corrections of presbyopia, common among them are shown in Flowchart 10.1.

Single Vision Lenses

The patient with emmetropia or low degree of hyperopia is usually very happy with single vision near spectacle. Single vision correction with near correction provides a wide field of view unmatched by any other lens form for presbyopia, but they cause blurring of distant vision. One option for patients without any effect on distance vision is half eye spectacles that allows them to look over the near vision lens and view distant objects clearly. Some patients who experience significant difficulty using multifocal lenses may also prefer to use separate pairs of glasses for distance and near. A single vision correction offers the advantage of a large, clear field of vision, and is also the least expensive option. This may be the option of choice for the new emergent presbyope. However, it is wise to avoid prescribing single vision lenses or separate pair to develop the habit of wearing near correction and appreciate bifocals later. By postponing, it is quite likely that near correction will be stronger with more optical difficulties and adaptive problems. However, they are a better solution in case of anisometropia, patients with orthopedic problems, or when the bifocals are refused for cosmetic reasons or prior poor performance.

Bifocal Lenses

Bifocal lenses (Fig. 10.1) incorporate the distance vision and the near vision prescriptions into a single spectacle lens. The majority of the lens area contains the distant vision correction while the near vision correction is confined to a smaller segment in the lower portion of the lens. The configuration allows the patient to alternate between distant lens portion and near lens portion. A variety of segment shapes and sizes are available and a selection may be made on the basis of their features and needs of the specific patient.

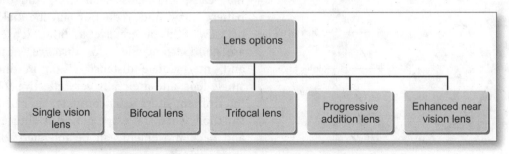

FLOWCHART 10.1: Lens options available for presbyopic patients

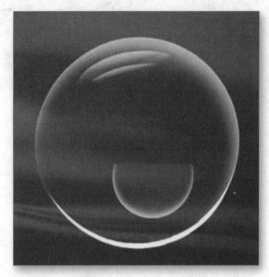

FIGURE 10.1: Bifocal lenses

Trifocal Lenses

Trifocal lenses (Fig. 10.2) incorporate distance, intermediate and near lens prescriptions, which is often important for patients who have advanced presbyopia. Trifocal lenses are also manufactured in variety of types and sizes. The option of an additional intermediate segment of these lenses may improve vision for the patient who is frequently involved in intermediate distance tasks. Trifocal lenses can be good for more advanced presbyopes who are intolerant to distant blur and require clear vision at their computer distance. These patient use bifocals or trifocals for their general wear and are averse to progressives or occupational enhanced near vision lens.

Progressive Addition Lenses

Progressive addition lenses are multifocal lens design used to correct presbyopia. These lenses are characterized by a smooth continuous change of power across the lens surface, with undesired zones that create vision distortions at the lower periphery. The power distribution and power transition in progressive lenses vary from one design to another. Relevant design parameters include length of the progressive corridor, size, shape and location of the near zone, transition between distance and near zones and asphericity. The smooth change in the power across the lens surface provides the user a region with intermediate power. It is for this reason they are most commonly prescribed for computer use. However, the region for intermediate power is like a very narrow valley. If the patient requires significant viewing at intermediate distance or spend most of his day on computer, he must continuously find the correct spot in the lens and use his neck to move the head rather than moving his eyes. This may cause musculoskeletal stress and the patient may find reduction in the field of view. Still progressive addition lenses are good arrangement for distance, near and intermediate distance vision in one single lens; and are really very effective for intermittent short-term computer user in a situation when the work period is shorter and neck movement can be tolerated for short period.

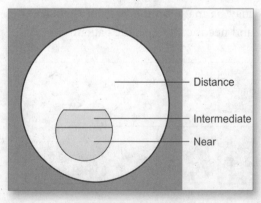

Distance

Intermediate

Near

FIGURE 10.2: Trifocal lenses

Enhanced Near Vision Lenses

Enhanced near vision lenses are specially designed lenses that meet the presbyopic demands of the patient's with extensive intermediate viewing needs such as computer users, assembly line workers, clerks, general office work, etc. The lens design provides a reasonably large intermediate vision on the top of the lens to enable the wearer to navigate the workplace. The magnitude of unwanted cylinder in occupational enhanced near vision lenses is significantly less than that in a progressive addition lenses because total power change is less, resulting in wider viewing zones compared to the progressive addition lens. However, they do not meet general viewing needs outside the workplace. Occupational enhanced near vision lenses can be very successful in meeting the occupational visual needs of most presbyopes.

CHALLENGES OF PRESBYOPIC DISPENSING

Presbyopia offers many challenges to the practitioner specially if the patient is visually demanding at near and extended near distance. A dynamic approach is needed to design a suitable correction for his occupational needs. Most common challenges associated with presbyopic optical dispensing are shown in the Flowchart 10.2.

Correction for Various Distances

Presbyopic difficulties for close works are not just the problem of near vision at 40 cm, but are a problem of reduced vision at various reading distances because the amount of accommodation used to maintain a clear vision varies with the distance of the object and it increases with decreasing distance. Patient satisfaction depends a lot on the lens type and patient subjective responses. The real difficulty is encountered while trying to correct the presbyopia for various distances. There is a need to trade-offs because of the limitations of optics. The optician needs to pick up the distance where there is a need to look at most often and then provide the suitable correction. The correction may be designed in single vision, bifocal or multifocal. The evolution of modern lens designs have increased the potential number of alternative options that can be dispensed successfully for full-time, part-time or just for occupational purposes. Modern offices using computers require more than one focusing point in a single pair lenses where single vision lenses may not work. The two distances can be selected based upon the visual needs of the wearer and a solution may be proposed. They might also be benefitted to use progressive addition lenses. Although progressive addition lenses

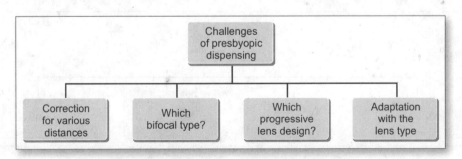

FLOWCHART 10.2: Challenges of presbyopic dispensing

provide distance, intermediate and near vision in one lens, it may not be perfect solution for extensive intermediate work. Extended near vision lens that provides a full reading prescription in the bottom half of the lens and a weakened prescription at the top for viewing a monitor, provide a preferred solution. Prescribing these lenses with an additional pair of general purpose progressive addition lens may be a conclusive solution. Similarly for a patient with a habit of reading in supine condition, a half eye reading lens with a general purpose progressive addition lens make a conclusive solution.

A progressive lens corrects vision not only at distance and near viewing distance but also at various intermediate distances. But it has its designing limitations. The straight forward meaning is there is no one single solution available for correcting presbyopia. A single pair lens cannot provide the comprehensive solution for today's lifestyle and all visual needs of presbyopic populations. Asking questions, understanding the visual needs, showing concerns about the needs and explaining how vision system is compromised if there is a compromised correction and finally providing the suitable solution are key. The solution may include one general purpose progressive addition lens and one occupational lens or it may include two separate distance and reading lenses together with one occupational lens or as needed.

Which Bifocal Lens Design?

Several types of bifocal lenses are available, selecting one among them needs some considerations on certain important factors as shown in Flowchart 10.3.

Image Jump

When looking from distance portion to the near portion of a bifocal lens, the sudden change in the prismatic effect because of the introduction of the base down prism by the near segment causes the world to "jump". The jump so noticed is very disturbing particularly with steps and kerbs. It has both vertical and horizontal element. Jump occurs all around the edge of the bifocal segment, although it is at the top part where it is most frequently noticed. The amount of jump is simply the magnitude of the prismatic effect exerted by the segment at its dividing line and is the product of the distance from the segment top to the segment optical center, in centimeters. For most of the E-style bifocal, with its distance and near optical

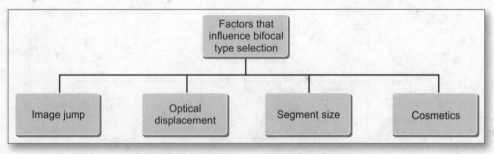

FLOWCHART 10.3: Factors affecting bifocal type selection

centers coinciding at the dividing line, the vertical jump is almost nil. Jump increases as the distance from the segment top to the segment optical center increases. It is less with flat-top segments and is more with round segments. The larger the segment is, the larger the effect of jump will be. To eliminate the jump effect in a bifocal lens, it is necessary to work the segment in such a manner that its optical center coincides with the segment top. The effect of jump is completely independent of the power of the main lens and the position of the distance optical center.

Optical Displacement

When a wearer gazes downward to read through the single vision lens he looks from a point that is away from the optical center of the lens, he encounters a prismatic effect as the object is appeared to shift towards apex. Or in other words, object is displaced away from the base of the prism towards its apex. The prismatic effect changes in the near visual zone when he wears a bifocal lens because bifocal lenses are made of two separate components—a main lens with a distance prescription and a supplementary segment lens with a power equal to reading addition. The distance optical center is at the center of the main lens and the near optical center is at the center of the near segment lens. They are separated by a distance depending upon the near segment design. The total power of the near portion is the sum of the distance portion power and the reading addition of the lens and the prismatic effect at some point in the near portion is given by the sum of the prismatic effect of the distance portion and the prismatic effect of the segment lens. Therefore the amount

of displacement of the object would be determined by sum of the prismatic effect of main lens and the segment lens.

In case of round shaped bifocal, base up prismatic effect would be exerted in plus lens prescription when a wearer would see from distance to near viewing point (NVP) and base down prismatic effect would be exerted because of near segment. The total prismatic effect would be the sum of the two prismatic effects. In case of a D-shape bifocal, assuming the NVP is located at the same point where optical center of the near segment is located, the net prismatic effect would be the result of the prismatic effect of the distance portion only. In case of E-style bifocal, the optical center of the segment is positioned on the diving line which is above the NVP. Since the power of the segment is positive, the segment will exert base up prism. Therefore, the total prismatic effect would be the sum of base up prismatic effect because of distance portion and base up prismatic effect because of near segment addition.

In case of minus power, the distance portion will exert base down prism. Consequently the prismatic effect will change depending upon the type of the segment shape. E-style bifocal will exert least prismatic effect in minus power. In case of straight top D-shape bifocal which has an optical center coinciding with the NVP, the vertical prismatic effect at reading level is due to the distance power only. Therefore it does not change when the wearer switches from single vision to bifocal lens. In case of round shaped bifocal base down prismatic effect would be exerted on minus lens power and base down prismatic effect would be exerted by near segment. The total prismatic effect would be the sum of the two prismatic effects.

Segment Size

The segment size determines the field of view through the near segment for a given vertex distance and pupil size. Occupational needs require the wider field of view at near distance because it is really irritating for many people to notice blur vision at the segment edge during quick eye movement laterally. Probably for this reason the larger near segments are gaining more popularity. Besides, occupational needs past habits of the wearer also determines the size of the near segment. A user of "E" style bifocal will always find it difficult to navigate during near vision task when he is switched to smaller size near segment lens. Wider segment size always minimizes head movement during excursion of eyes while reading and minimizes fatigue. One of the guidelines that can be helpful for size selection for near segment may be given as size is proportional to the percentage of time the lens is used for near work. Meaning a person who is engaged more in near task needs larger near segment than a person who does not have reading task. An avid reader may be benefitted more with wider near segment than most other people. During peripheral vision eyes move round the center of rotation and the line of sight makes an angle to the optical axis upto 30° as the wearer observes the objects in the visual field. Within this area the eye movement may not be in unison with lens movement. A round segment size of 20 mm provides macular field of view to the tune of approximately 35° in all direction for a vertex distance of 13 mm and center of rotation of the eye located at 14 mm behind the corneal apex.

Cosmetics

The conspicuous diving line is least visible in round segmented bifocal lenses and is most prominently visible in E-style bifocal. Most people like to choose one that is least appealing to ensure maximum cosmetic value.

Which Progressive Lens Design?

Progressive addition lenses are one piece lenses that vary gradually in surface curvature from a minimum value in the upper distance portion to a maximum value in the lower near portion. The upper portion of the lens provides the necessary distance correction, and the lower portion of the lens provides near correction. The 2 portions of the lens are connected seamlessly providing the wearer with a continuous depth of field from near to far. The increased power is achieved by constantly changing radius of curvature from distance portion to near portion. Change in radius of curvature results in surface astigmatism at the temporal and nasal side of the lens. Surface astigmatism produces an unwanted cylinder error that blurs vision and limits the wearer's field of clear vision. The wearer gets following advantages over segmented multifocal lenses:

1. No line of demarcation provides more cosmetically appealing lens with continuous vision, free from visually distracting borders. The lens looks like a single vision lens.

2. Progressive addition lens offers a greater visual flexibility with uninterrupted clear vision from distance to near. At virtually every point the eye finds the appropriate lens power that matches for

the distance at which it is focusing. This is an additional visual advantage over conventional bifocal lenses.

3. Unlike conventional bifocal lens, the progressive lens does not produce any image jump when the eyes move from distance viewing zone to near viewing zone or vice versa.

Above-mentioned 3 attributes of progressive addition lenses are strong message communicator to allure any one to opt for a progressive lens. They also make the life of the optician easy to dispense progressive lenses. Probably this is the reason why more than 75 million people are now using progressive lenses successfully. However, the above features of the progressive addition lenses provide huge progressive design possibility:

1. Changes in curvature profile from minimum value to maximum value may differ providing various progressive lens design possibilities with respect to the length and width of different viewing zones.

2. The magnitude and rate of change in unwanted cylinder in the lateral blending region that causes image swim, skew distortion and other optical side effects may differ.

3. The distribution and orientation of cylinder power may also impact design changes.

4. The progressive curves may be on the front surface or back surface of the lens or may have its progressive components split between the front and back surfaces of the lens.

These design factors differentiate one progressive lens from the other. When a dispensing optician opens the list of the progressive lens menu, he finds himself lost in the sea of confusion. Moreover, the lens manufacturers do not even release the true technical information about design features. Most of the information available from lens manufacturer is in the form of information bulletin designed to attract the actual users. Different lens manufacturer uses different terminologies that also makes it difficult to compare one progressive lens design to another. The dispensing opticians do not have instruments to check the progressive lens design and identify the most suitable one in their dispensary because of unavailability and cost. Complicating the matter is the positioning of different progressive lens designs. Each new design is introduced with one unique feature and is placed at a higher price bracket than the previous one. Justifying the price factor is also an issue for the dispensing optician. Hard design concentrates the progressive optics into the smaller regions of the lens surface, thereby increasing the magnitude of unwanted cylinder and the progressive gradients. It provides wider distance and near viewing zones, but higher levels of blur and distortion in the periphery. It is good for sustained viewing task either at distance or at near, requiring good visual acuity. It tends to offer the similar utility that current bifocal wearer enjoys and increases cosmetic acceptance. Soft design spreads the progressive optics across larger regions of the lens surface, thereby reducing the gradients and overall unwanted cylinder at the expense of narrowing the areas of clear vision. It is good for dynamic viewing tasks and it tends to improve visual comfort and adaptation. The new generations progressive lens designs are highly technologically driven. They have more complicated design features. Putting them so simply would be misnomer. The new "free form lens" surfacing process can produce complex surfaces with exceptional accuracy and smoothness using 3-axis generator. The surface is cut not only in vertical and horizontal direction, but it is also cut following the spiral cutting path to optimize the lens surface to fine tune the optical performance of the lenses on eyes by customizing them taking additional information like frame shapes, frame sizes and nonstandard frame curves. The process allows the optics of the lens design to take full advantage of the available lens area. Significant difference is noted in the optical performance of the lenses as perceived by the wearer. It improves the real life optical performance of the central viewing region of the lens. Lifestyle customization including biometrical data aims to match the optics of the lens design to wearer's occupational needs and is tailored to wearer so that the lens adapts to him. With so many options available the optician needs to consider more while dispensing progressive lenses and also needs some tools that allow matching the lens design to the wearer's visual needs.

Adaptation with the Lens Type

Presbyopia is an irreversible condition and is an evolutionary blunder that comes as a psychological shock to a person. The person starts facing difficulties in near and extended near vision task that grow gradually and have multiple effects on quality of life. The condition brings in lot of adaptive changes in the person. He develops the habit of squinting at the reading material and starts

extending his hands to read. Some people find it more easy to take their head posture back to read comfortably. If the condition remains untreated for a longer period of time, it causes significant functional visual disability. When the correction is used in the form of multifocal lenses, the wearer needs to make some adaptation to develop new visual habits in the new visual environment.

An emmetrope or a person who wears only single vision lenses, he generally turns his head up to look at distance and turns his head slightly down to look at near vision task. When he uses the bifocal lenses he needs to break this habit and develop the habit of keeping the head straight and depress the eye to look at near vision task and turn the head slightly down to look at distance through the top portion of the bifocal lenses. This is because if he turns his head down he will push the near viewing zone further down and while viewing at distance if he turns his head up he will find the top arc line of the near segment obstructing distance viewing.

A bifocal or a multifocal lens contains two or more zones for viewing at multiple distances. Many a times a wearer finds it difficult to find the right portion to look at a particular distance. This is very common in progressive lenses as different viewing zones are seamlessly combined together. The difficulty is minimized over a period of time and the wearer starts finding the right zone after the initial period of adaptation.

Another adaptation that a new wearer has to do with his new bifocal or multifocal lenses is to change his head and eye movement during reading. He finds himself not being able to read full width of the line. He needs to learn to move his head while doing his near viewing task. In order to keep the optics of the lens clear and maintain the line of sight through the center of the near segment, he needs to co-ordinate the head and eye movement during near vision task. Some patients also feel swimming sensation or warped appearance of line during lateral eye movement. A lot of patients find it difficult while going up and down on staircase with their bifocal lenses. Sometimes they find floor out of focus when they look through the near segment; while other times they find the dividing line interfering with their vision. They need to learn to turn their head down more than they usually do so that they look over the top of the bifocal area.

Adapting to new lens type requires a patient to break his visual habits of past and develop a new that complement with the new mode of vision correction. The first time user may have some unusual sensations and may feel:

- The presence of demarcation line.
- When he walks or moves his head rapidly, objects to the side may appear to move slightly.

These sensations will disappear quickly with continued use and the patient will soon have the most natural vision possible. The shortest and surest way to adapt is to continue wearing them with intermittent removal for short duration if he feels temporary difficulties. The eyes will find the right area swiftly and naturally. However, the length of time needed for adaptation is subjective. While some people are lucky who get adapted very fast, many people take time. The process is similar to break into a new pair of shoes. One of the simplest ways is to use the new bifocal lenses in small doses. Use only while reading during the initial days to appreciate the new lens type, and you will gradually find yourself more and more able to use bifocal lenses. Although this prolongs the adaptation period, the wearer finds it easier to adapt. Of course the quicker way is to wear them all the time. Some of the tips that can be explained to the wearer to adapt easily and quickly are:

1. Stop thinking that you are using bifocal lenses.
2. If you see blur from the bottom, avoid seeing the floor from the bottom.
3. Do not pay attention to any unusual sensation.
4. When you find it too difficult, remove the spectacle and relax for a few minutes before putting them on again.
5. Spend some days patiently to use bifocal lenses. You may refrain from using while moving.
6. Even after using it for some days, if it does not suit visit your optician and consult them again.

Adaptation issues can be managed well by educating the patient. The educated consumer will be your best customer. Help your patient to understand their visual problems and the solutions you have to offer. Explain adaptation verbally before and after dispensing, and supply written instructions to reinforce the information. The better the patient understands what he will need to adjust, the better the chances of successful adaptation. It is important that before putting a patient into an adaptation period, you must explain the patient what an adaptation period is likely to be and how will you help him when the adaptation period is over. Most important is you need to bring the patient into your confidence. Millions of people wear bifocals or progressive lenses successfully and the patient will soon be one of them. Explain them to accept the idea of wearing bifocals. Keep in mind that the bifocal reading segment provides sharp vision at a specific distance range from one's eyes. An object lying outside the range on either side will be blurred, so the patient may have to move either closer or farther from that object to see it clearly. Having a difficult or slow time adjusting to bifocals does not mean that a mistake was made. Of course, errors can happen, but 99% of the time it is simply a matter of adapting to the new lens type. If a person has been diligent in trying them for a few weeks and still thinks the lenses are not right, must have the dispensing optician check them again.

POINTS TO REMEMBER

- Presbyopia is not just the problem of near vision at 40 cm, but is a problem of reduced vision at various reading distances.
- When looking from distance portion to the near portion of a bifocal lens, the sudden change in the prismatic effect because of the introduction of the base down prism by the segment causes the world "jump".
- Image jump produced by segmented bifocal lenses is least with "E" style bifocal lenses.
- Optical displacement produced by segmented bifocal lenses is lens power dependent.
- Unlike conventional bifocal lenses, the progressive lens does not produce any image jump when the eyes move from distance viewing zone to near viewing zone or vice versa.

CHAPTER 11

PROGRESSIVE ADDITION LENS DISPENSING

Progressive addition lenses are also known as "no line multifocal lenses". The lenses provide better vision solution than traditional bifocals. Instead of having just 2 lens powers like a bifocal—one for distance vision and the other for up-close—progressive lenses have a gradual change in power from the top to the bottom of the lens, providing a range of powers for clear vision for long distance, up-close and everywhere in between. Progressive lenses provide the closest to natural vision after the onset of presbyopia. While progressive lenses are currently the most popular correction option, dispensing progressive lenses are still a nightmare for many opticians. Choosing the right frame for progressive lens, choosing the right progressive lens design and measuring dispensing parameters — all are critical. Chapter 11 is compiled with an objective to discuss dispensing progressive addition lenses and challenges associated with it.

Progressive addition lenses are primarily used in the treatment of presbyopic patients who are normally above the age of 40 years. Until early 1980s almost all multifocal lenses dispensed were segmented bifocal and trifocal type. Since then there had been a steady growth in the usage of progressive addition lenses and today more than 50% of multifocal lenses dispensed across the world are progressive addition lenses. Several studies have shown that a large percentage of patients prefer progressive lenses over segmented multifocal lenses for 4 driving factors. These driving factors are strong enough to provide an edge over segmented multifocal lenses to the patients. They are:

1. No demarcation line.
2. No image jump when the vision shifts from distance to near and vice versa.
3. Continuous field of clear vision from near to distance, providing correct power for every distance from near to long distance.
4. Helps negotiating staircases with minimum head bend.

Moreover, there is a detracting feature of progressive lens, i.e. the lens design results in unwanted cylinder in the periphery of the lens, usually located in the lower temporal and nasal portion of the lens. This unique lens designing process of progressive addition lenses provides a lens with 4 important zones as shown in Figure 11.1.

1. Distance viewing zone of the progressive lenses is located on the superior half of the lens.
2. The stabilized near viewing zone of the progressive lenses is located at the lower half that provides the specified near add power for reading.
3. A progressive corridor that connects the distance and near zones providing a zone that allows looking at various mid-range vision.
4. The 2 blending regions located at lower temporal and nasal portion of the lens produce blur and distortion and offer only minimal visual utility.

PROGRESSIVE ADDITION LENS REFERENCE MARKINGS

The typical surface geometry of progressive addition lens is entirely with no visible reference marks. It is, for this reason all the manufacturers provide some reference markings. These reference markings facilitate lens positioning, lens processing and lens verification during dispensing. Understanding these reference markings are critical to successful dispensing of progressive addition lenses. Broadly there are 2 sets of markings on all progressive addition lenses as shown in Table 11.1.

Table 11.1:

Progressive addition lens markings	
Permanent markings	*Temporary markings*
Alignment reference circles	Prism reference point
Near addition	Fitting cross
Brand logo	Distance power circle
	Near power circle

Permanent Markings

Permanent markings are irremovable laser markings on the lens that are engraved and located on nonusable area of the lens. When the ink marking is removed, they are made visible by fogging the lens or by using specially designed tools known as

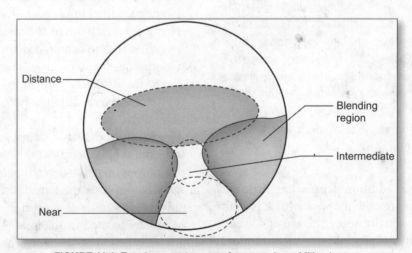

FIGURE 11.1: Four important zones of progressive addition lenses

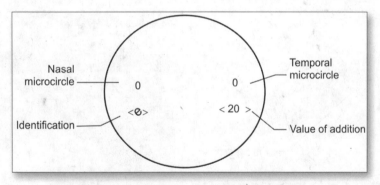

FIGURE 11.2: Permanent markings of progressive addition lenses

PAL ID. Two small hidden engravings are permanently etched at 17 mm on either side of the prism reference point (PRP), i.e. they are 34 mm apart on the horizontal line. They are the basis for remarking according to the template of the progressive lens design. Figure 11.2 shows the two hidden circles. Brand logo is mostly engraved below the nasal hidden circle and the near addition is below the temporal hidden circle.

Temporary Markings

Temporary markings are ink markings on the lens. They are removed prior to lens wear. These markings are very important for lens dispensing and are always utilized to position the lens during lens glazing, lens fitting and verifications. The temporary markings are shown in Flowchart 11.1.

Geometrical Center

Figure 11.3 shows the geometrical center of the lens lying at the midpoint of the horizontal center line. Umbilical line also

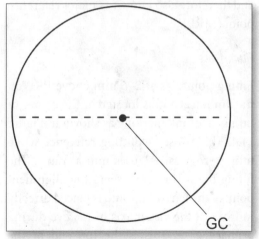

FIGURE 11.3: Geometrical center of progressive addition lens

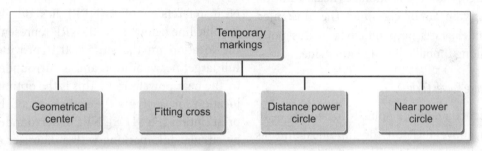

FLOWCHART 11.1: Temporary ink markings

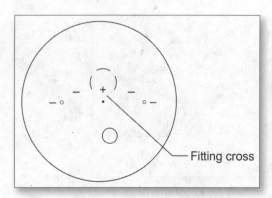

FIGURE 11.4: Fitting cross

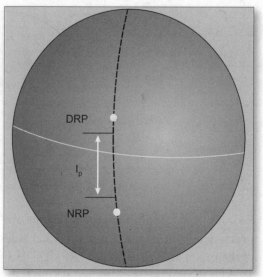

FIGURE 11.5: Distance reference point and near reference point

passes through it. This is also known as prism reference point (PRP) that is used to check the prism in the lens. This is also the distance optical center (DOC) of the lens, and therefore also known as major reference point (MRP).

Fitting Cross

Fitting point lies at 2–6 mm above PRP on the umbilical and is located at the center of fitting cross ink marking as shown in Figure 11.4. This is used as fitting reference while fitting progressive lenses into a frame. The fitting point (FP) represents the alignment point of the lens design and is placed directly in front of the visual axis of the eye during primary gaze. This is the top end of the corridor length from where curvature starts changing to accommodate near addition along the umbilical line. The unwanted cylinder starts perpendicular to this point all along umbillic line on either side.

Distance Power Circle

Distance reference point is located at 6–10 mm above PRP on the umbilical line as shown in Figure 11.5. The distance reference

point (DRP) represents the location on the surface that provides the exact base curve and is the optimal location for verifying the distance prescription. Distance power circle surrounds the DRP by circular ink marking which is usually 10–15 mm in diameter. Most often this appears as half circle to ensure a reasonable distance from the fitting cross. The location of DRP is somewhat arbitrary; it is generally located to ensure error-free verification of the prescription.

Near Power Circle

Near reference point (NRP) lies on the umbilic line below the PRP. NRP represents the location on the surface that provides full target near addition and is surrounded by the near power circle. This is the optimal location for verifying the add power of the prescription (Fig. 11.5). NRP is surrounded by circular ink marking with a diameter of 8 mm or more. The circle denotes stable spherical near zone. The top edge of this circle on umbilic line is commonly taken as the end point of progressive corridor length, where 85% of near addition is achieved depending upon design philosophy.

IDEAL FRAME SELECTION

The key to success in progressive lens dispensing is judicious selection of spectacle frame, correct selection of corridor length of the progressive addition lens and, taking the required dispensing measurements accurately and effectively. While selecting the frame for progressive lenses make sure that the shape of the frame allows for minimum fitting height for the recommended progressive lens design and also allows for sufficient amount of clearance above the fitting cross as shown in Figure 11.6.

The 2 most important factors to pay attention are shown in the Flowchart 11.2:

Shape of the Frame

The symmetrical frame shape where the difference between "A" measurement and "B" measurement is not significant, as nearest to ideal frame shape is for progressive lens dispensing. Figure 11.7 shows the various shapes of the frames. Square and panto shapes are the most suitable shapes for the progressive addition lenses. Steep rectangular shapes that extend beyond the temporal bone of the face may not be suitable. Aviator shape reduces the size of the reading area by being too "cut away" in the nasal area of the frame which may be contraindicated when the pupillary distance is narrow.

Size/Depth of the Frame

The selected frame must have sufficient depth to accommodate the entire zones of the progressive lens from the top of the

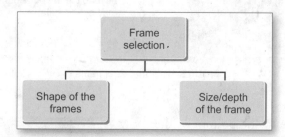

FLOWCHART 11.2: Two important factors for ideal frame selection

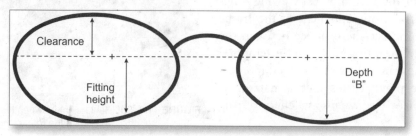

FIGURE 11.6: Ideal frame geometry for progressive addition lenses

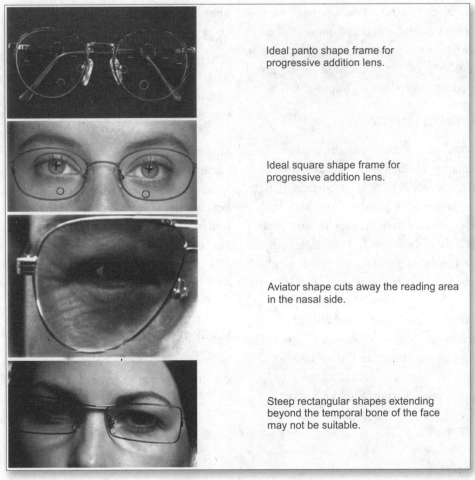

Ideal panto shape frame for progressive addition lens.

Ideal square shape frame for progressive addition lens.

Aviator shape cuts away the reading area in the nasal side.

Steep rectangular shapes extending beyond the temporal bone of the face may not be suitable.

FIGURE 11.7: Shapes of frame

distance power circle to the bottom of the near power circle within its lens aperture, i.e. the "B" measurement should be enough to include full distance and near viewing zones (Fig. 11.8). "A" measurement of the frame should minimize the distance between the position of the fitting cross and the temporal end of the frame eyewire. This is important when the pupillary distance is narrow as it minimizes the swimming effect during lateral gaze.

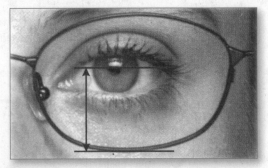

FIGURE 11.8: Sufficient height between the pupil and the lower rim of the frame

CORRIDOR LENGTH SELECTION

Corridor length of the progressive addition lens defines the section on the umbilical line that features gradual change in base curve from a minimum value to value that is 85% of the maximum value (Fig. 11.9). The top end of the corridor length is at the center of fitting cross and the bottom end of the corridor length is at the point where 85% of the near addition is achieved. This is usually achieved at the top edge of the near power circle depending upon lens design. The

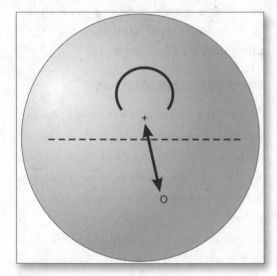

FIGURE 11.9: Corridor length of progressive addition lenses

length of the corridor may vary between 10–21 mm or more depending upon specific lens design. A shorter corridor length implies that the optics of lens design is compressed, due to mathematical constraints of progressive lens design that increases the rate of change in unwanted cylinder across the lens design, leading to narrower central viewing zone and reduced intermediate utility. The wearer may also feel more swimming effect during lateral head and eye movement. Ultimately adaptation to lens may remain an issue. On the contrary longer corridor length implies that the wearer needs larger down gaze eye rotation to reach full strength near addition or if the "B" measurement of the frame is smaller near viewing zone may cut away. Ultimately reading vision may be an issue. The straight forward meaning is an appropriate corridor length selection is the key to successful progressive lens dispensing and it should be based upon several factors as mentioned in the Flowchart 11.3.

Frame Selection

The selected frame is perhaps the most immediately noticed factor while selecting the corridor length of the progressive

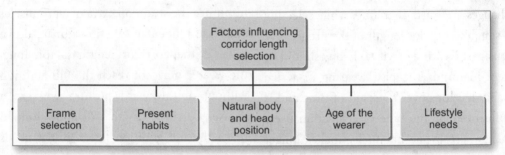

FLOWCHART 11.3: Factors for corridor length selection

addition lens. Unless the corridor length required by "B" measurement of the frame is matched adequately, the wearer will have to tolerate the unnecessary optical compromise. The objective is to match the optics of the lens design to maximize the near utility of the lens based upon fitting height measurements so that the wearer can enjoy full advantage of the available lens area. Refer to Figure 11.6 that demonstrate the "B" measurement of the selected frame for progressive lenses must allow for minimum fitting height for the recommended progressive lens design below the fitting cross marking, and at the same time it also allows for sufficient amount of clearance above the fitting cross to accommodate complete area of distance power circle.

Present Habits

Knowing the present habits of the wearer is important in making smooth transitions through the adaptation period with the new progressive lenses. Getting used to a new multifocal or a new lens per se requires the patient to break his visual habits of past. It is always easier to adapt to a new lens when changes are least. Therefore, while selecting a suitable corridor length of the progressive lens past wearing or visual habits should be kept in mind. The past wearing or visual habit develops over a period of time and is influenced by the type of correction used. A new presbyope habitually makes longer head rotation during down gaze reading. It

implies that a longer corridor progressive lens design is better option for a new presbyope, if provided by other factors. On the contrary, a matured presbyope learns to reduce the head rotation angle and develops the habit of increased angle of ocular rotation over the years. He may be more benefitted with shorter corridor length, if provided by other factors. A user of round shaped bifocal lens would be benefitted with longer corridor length, whereas a user of Univis D bifocal would be more comfortable with shorter corridor length progressive lens design. A user of progressive addition lens should be given same corridor length unless otherwise indicated.

Natural Body and Head Position

The wearer's natural body and head position determines the vertical rotation of the eye for near and distance vision. The vertical position of near viewing zone influences the degree of down gaze required to view through the near addition. A well-designed progressive lens will always aim to establish the natural habit so as to place the near zone as high as possible that will minimize the amount of down gaze needed, and thereby minimize the strain on extra ocular muscles and ease binocular function during down gaze. If the corridor length is too long, the wearer may not reach the full addition without an awkward posture whereas a shorter corridor length will allow him to reach the full addition faster. But it needs a compensatory head positioning. The corridor length should be no shorter or longer than necessary. It must be within the limits of physiological comfortable vision which may be achieved in locating the usable near vision at down gaze position of about 22°–25°. Some researchers' opinion are 16 mm of corridor length represents the maximum length suitable for physiological comfortable vision. Every additional 1 mm of corridor length requires roughly 2° of additional down gaze ocular rotation.

Age of the Wearer

The wearer's age also influences corridor length selection for the progressive lenses. Early presbyope can accommodate for intermediate distance and can adjust their head position, whereas aging eyes can no longer accommodate to compensate for the lack of intermediate lens power. They should be more benefitted with little larger corridor length as permitted by other factors. However, a matured presbyope who had been using segmented bifocal lenses when switched to progressive lenses should be given shorter corridor length progressive lens so as to enable him to use it as bifocal lens.

Lifestyle Needs

The unique visual needs of the wearer specific to his lifestyle may also influence the choice of corridor length for progressive lens. Understanding lifestyle needs implies assessing the relative visual demands and placing more importance to it minimizing

the immediate dissatisfaction. Relevant lifestyle information may be captured by asking questions and a suitable corridor length may be selected that provides the most suitable viewing zone configuration for the wearer, as permitted by other factors. Progressive lens wearers who are more frequently engaged in tasks associated with far vision would be more happy with larger corridor length progressive lens that provide smooth transition of near addition from minimum to maximum, whereas wearer with greater near vision demand would be happy if his down gaze vision reaches faster to full extent near addition.

The new backside progressive lens design configuration implies that the progressive power zones are closer to the eye than the front side progressive lens design. It implies that line of sight will reach the NRP quicker than that with front side progressive lens design. Therefore, the choice for corridor length has to be little shorter in order to allow the same position of near zone with respect to eye movement. There are 2 associated factors that also need to be considered while deciding upon the selection of the corridor length of the progressive lens design. They are:

- Minimum fitting height
- Recommended fitting height.

The underlying objective is to accommodate the full strength of near addition power and to ensure sufficient depth while reading. Minimum fitting

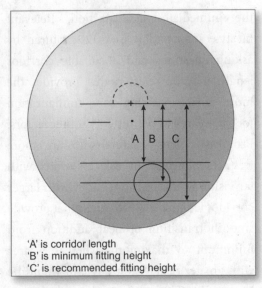

'A' is corridor length
'B' is minimum fitting height
'C' is recommended fitting height

FIGURE 11.10: Recommended fitting height

height lies at NRP where 100% near addition is achieved and recommended fitting height lies at the bottom end of the near power circle. If the fitting height allows to accommodate recommended fitting height as shown in the Figure 11.10 within the frame shape, the patient will enjoy good depth of vision while reading.

FITTING CROSS HEIGHT

The fitting cross ink marking is used as fitting reference while progressive lens

dispensing. The fitting point (FP) represents the alignment point of the lens design, which is to be placed directly in front of the visual axis of the eye in primary gaze. In order to place fitting cross at a designated place, the dispensing optician has to take necessary measurements. Flowchart 11.4 shows the 2-step process for measuring fitting cross height while dispensing progressive lenses.

Adjusting the Frame

Before you start measuring for fitting height it is important that you fit the selected frame on the wearer's face and then take the measurement. This is important as it provides stability of frame on wearer's face and makes sure that the position is not changed even after adjusting the frame on the wearer's face. The spectacle frame needs to be adjusted with respect to various aspects of frame fitting as shown in Flowchart 11.5.

Pantoscopic Angle

Pantoscopic angle implies that the top of the frame front lies away from the eyebrows and the bottom of the frame front moves

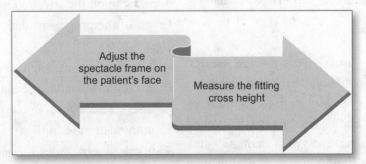

Adjust the spectacle frame on the patient's face

Measure the fitting cross height

FLOWCHART 11.4: Fitting height measuring procedure

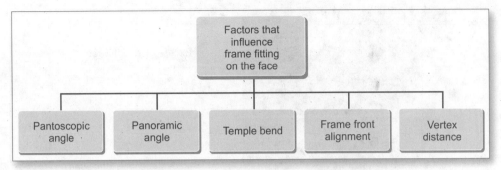

FLOWCHART 11.5: Important aspects of frame fitting

towards the cheeks, creating a parallel relation with facial plane as shown in Figure 11.11. It determines the vertical position of the fitting cross height on the wearer's face. It also divides the frame front on the wearer's face into 2 segments—the upper being used for distance vision and the lower being used for near vision. Thus it brings the near zone closer to the eyes and increases the field of view through the near zone of the lens. Pantoscopic tilt also minimizes the vertex distance changes and determines the vertical position of the frame front on the wearer's face. Fitting cross height should always be measured when the adequate

pantoscopic angle has been given to ensure correct vertical position of the frame front to minimize the probable error that may occur post fitting of lenses into the frame.

Panoramic Angle

Panoramic angle is the face form wrap of the spectacle frame front as shown in Figure 11.12. It ensures that the frame front follows the line of the wearer's face as seen from the top. It determines the angle at which the horizontal plane of the lens lies in relation to the horizontal plane of the face. Positive face form wrap is desired in which case the frame front sits slightly more forward from the

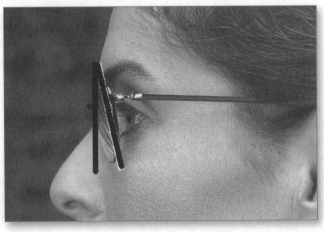

FIGURE 11.11: Pantoscopic tilt

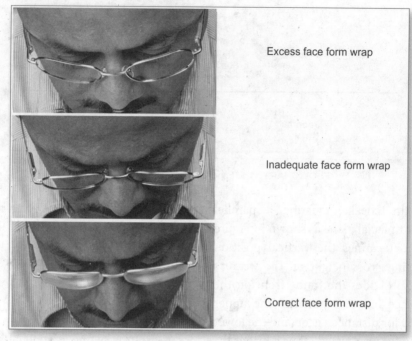

Excess face form wrap

Inadequate face form wrap

Correct face form wrap

FIGURE 11.12: Face form wrap

bridge than the end pieces of the frame. This is essential for both cosmetic and optical reasons as it brings the geometrical center of the frame nearer to the wearer's pupillary distance. Panoramic angle influences the horizontal position of the fitting cross. It is, therefore, prudent to fit the frame for panoramic tilt before measuring fitting cross height.

Temple Bend

In hockey end temple frame temple length determines the position on the temple from where it is bent to lock the frame from behind the ears and provide stability on the face (Fig. 11.13). Inadequate temple bend leads to instable frame and excess temple bend leads to increase in effective pantoscopic tilt on the wearer's face. Both are contraindicated for accurate fitting cross height measurement. It is, therefore, prudent to adjust temple length before measuring fitting cross height.

Frame Front Alignment

The spectacle frame must sit squarely on the face before measuring the fitting cross height. Adjust the angle of the temples and front alignment and then measure fitting cross height (Fig. 11.14). This is important to ensure that both eyes measurements for fitting cross height have been taken correctly. Sometimes it is quite likely that the position of the fitting cross is at different vertical position. Measuring fitting cross height after frame front alignment, it is possible to rule out the error and ensure that the difference in height is not because of fitting error but because of anatomical reasons.

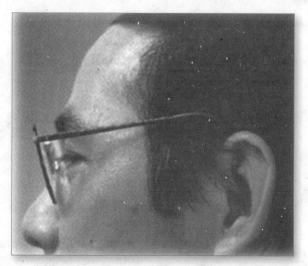

FIGURE 11.13: Needs to lengthen side bend

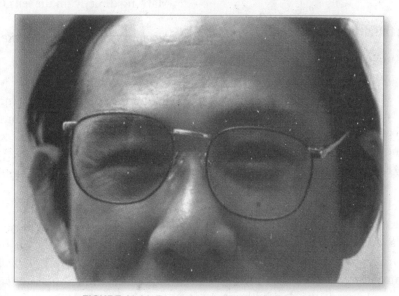

FIGURE 11.14: Front of the frame not in alignment

Vertex Distance

Vertex distance is the distance from the center of the back surface of the lens to the apex of the cornea as shown in Figure 11.15. In metal frames with adjustable nose pads vertex distance changes can be done by changing the angles of the nose pads. This is not possible with the plastic frame, in which case temple bend determines the frame stability and corresponding vertex distance. Measuring the fitting cross height at correct vertex distance ensures the correct vertical measurement of fitting cross height.

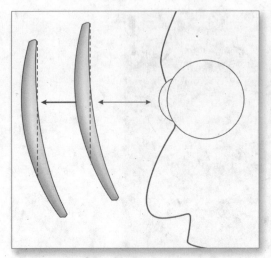

FIGURE 11.15: Vertex distance changes vertical location of fitting cross

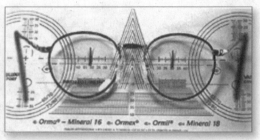

FIGURE 11.16: Using progressive lens layout card to mark monocular PD for distance

Measuring the Fitting Cross Height

Once all the above fitting adjustments are done and the frame is stable at the desired position, the correct positions of the fitting cross can be determined with respect to the horizontal and vertical location of the fitting cross in the frame of reference. Horizontal location of the fitting cross has to be matched with monocular PD for distance vision and the vertical position of the fitting cross is determined by the vertical distance between the centers of the pupil to lower rim of the spectacle frame front. The position where the 2 points intersects with each other with respect to the frame is the desired location where the fitting point of the progressive lens would be placed while fixing the lens into the given frame. Since fitting point is the alignment point for the progressive lens design, the correct placement of fitting point would mean that all the invisible zones of the progressive lens design would assume their desired positions and the visual axis of

the patient would coincide with optical axis of the lens in the primary gaze. There are 2 methods commonly practiced to measure fitting cross height:

1. Measuring monocular pupillary distance
2. Marking directly on the lens insert.

Measuring Monocular Pupillary Distance

There are different ways of measuring monocular PD for distance vision; the detailed procedure is explained in the Chapter 6. Once the monocular PD for distance is determined, mark their location on the lens insert by placing the frame symmetrically and aligning on the progressive addition lens layout card as shown in Figure 11.16. Mark a vertical line on each lens insert at the determined PD and place the frame back on the wearer's face to check the accuracy of PD. If the PD is correct, put the horizontal line mark across the marked vertical line so as to coincide with the pupil center height.

Now use the correct layout card of the selected lens design and place the frame with fitting cross marked on lens insert; coinciding with the fitting cross on the respective layout card and make sure that the full distance and near circles are within the frame rim as shown in Figure 11.17.

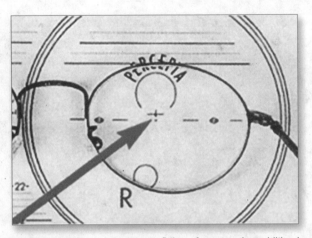

FIGURE 11.17: Using layout card to ensure proper fitting of progressive addition lens into frame

Finally, put on the frame on the wearer's face and again make sure that the fitting cross on progressive addition lens must coincide with the pupil center of the wearer in their natural posture and measure the fitting height as shown in Figure 11.18. The fitting height is specified in millimeter as the distance above the deepest point of the inner frame rim to the intersection point of cross marking on lens insert.

Marking Directly on the Lens Insert

This is the single step method of measuring the fitting cross height as shown in the Figure 11.19.

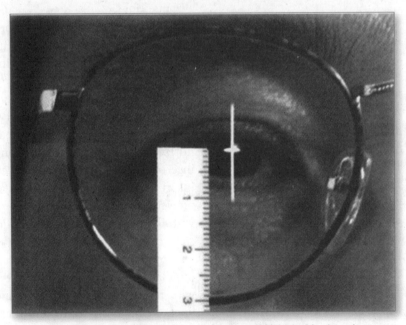

FIGURE 11.18: Fitting height measurement (29 mm in this picture)

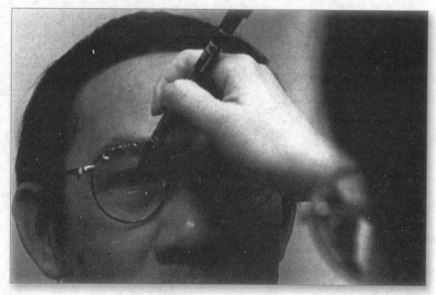

FIGURE 11.19: Fitting cross height marking on lens insert

1. Ask the patient to take a stable position and then place yourself opposite and at the same height as that of the patient.
2. Ask him to look straight ahead to your right eye.
3. Hold a pen torch just below your right eye.
4. Close your left eye to avoid parallax error.
5. Observe the position of the light reflex in the patient's left eye.
6. Place a small dot mark on the lens insert corresponding to the pupil reflex.
7. Ask the patient to look at your left eye and complete the procedure for the other eye.
8. Remove the frame, put it face down on the cross chart such that the dot coincides with the intersection of the cross.
9. Mark the fitting cross on the lens insert, place the frame again on the patient's face and check the correctness of the marking.
10. Move the frame up and down slightly, let it settle, and recheck for both eyes markings.
11. Finally, measure the fitting height from the center of the cross to the deepest point of the inner frame rim on lens insert.

Some opticians are unable to mark directly on the lens insert when the frame is on the wearer's face. They may draw 2 horizontal and vertical lines on the lens insert so that they divide the entire lens insert into 4 quadrants. Now put the frame on wearer's face and observe the pupil reflex with the respect to quadrant. Following the steps from 1 to 5 as mentioned above make an approximation of the location of the pupillary reflex observed in the quadrant with respect to the horizontal and vertical lines. Remove the frame and mark the dot on lens insert. Put the frame back on the

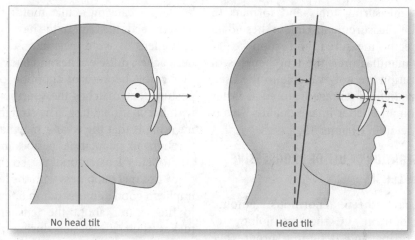

No head tilt

Head tilt

FIGURE 11.20: Head tilt results in error while measuring fitting cross height

face and reverify the position of the dot and if needed make necessary corrections in dot position. Finally, mark fitting cross and measure the fitting height from the center of the cross to the deepest point of the inner frame rim on lens insert. The method provides a reference for marking that minimizes the possibility of error.

Measuring the height of fitting cross is very critical for successful dispensing of the progressive addition lenses. Hence care must be taken to ensure that the patient assumes his habitual head posture because any typical head tilt will result in significant fitting height measurement errors (Fig. 11.20).

DISPENSING CUSTOMIZED PROGRESSIVE ADDITION LENSES

The introduction of new free-form technology in lens manufacturing has brought 2 major changes in progressive lens designing. The progressive design has been brought to back surface of the lens which means the viewing corridors are closer to the eyes. This reduces the magnification effect over the entire viewing zones of rear side progressive lens. The advantage is noticed in the lens periphery and disadvantage is noticed in reading zone. Less magnification differences means less distortion and less swimming effect. Less magnification also means smaller letters could mislead the patient to want the higher addition which is not the good idea for all the known reasons. It also means that the patient's eyes would reach faster to near viewing zone to read, so corridor length has to be adjusted in order to allow the same positioning of near zone with respect to eye movement. Another advantage of the new technology is that the optics of actual lens is fine tuned on point-by-point basis using complex aspherization algorithms until the final lens produces the desired optical performance of the target lens as closely as possible. The new customized progressive lenses need some additional dispensing measurements to be supplied to the lens laboratories. These data are incorporated while lens designing to minimize the errors and improve the lens performance. Lens manufacturer provides measuring tools and formats to record the measurement. Unless these data are correctly measured and supplied to the lens manufacturer, the true benefits of customization are not available to the user. The immediate advantage is noted as faster adaptation and better image quality. This is dealt in detail in Chapter 15.

DEMONSTRATION OF USE OF PROGRESSIVE ADDITION LENSES

There have been enormous amount of development in the technology of manufacturing and designing progressive addition lens surface. Still it is impossible to design progressive lens surface without optical error in the periphery of the lens that limits the width of the usable areas. The complicated surface geometry coupled with invisible viewing zones creates a situation where a small number of the wearer finds themselves hunting for the right place to look through, resulting in dissatisfactions. This is because of the nonadaptation to the lenses. Adapting to the new progressive lens requires that the wearer must move his head appropriately for distance and near viewing zones, i.e. upwards for near and downwards for distance. This is exactly opposite to the way to which a nonpresbyope is accustomed to. Some wearer feels instability initially while walking or on staircase because of the constant search for the small intermediate viewing zone. There are some wearers who may complain of having to move their head from side to side to read the complete size of the text. Another adaptation issue is "swim effect" that is apparent in dynamic situation when the wearer makes lateral eye movement. The wearer can report dizziness, nausea or physical distress because of swim effect. There are comfort issues which may be because of unequal prism thinning between right and left lenses causing ocular motor stress. The wearer needs to adapt to the new ergonomics of the lens to avoid frustrations with vision, neck aches, muscle aches and back aches that may result because of adoption of unusual posture that matches the specific lens zone with occupational task. The straight forward meaning is that the wearer may have to pass through an adaptation period in order to attain better lens ergonomics so that he can enjoy optimal happiness with the lenses. This implies a good demonstration or explanation to the wearer about the lens ergonomics makes their life easier during adaptation period. A good demonstration of progressive addition lens usage follows a sequential process that starts with demonstrating the distance vision.

1. Put the spectacle on the wearer's face and ask him to tilt his head down so that he looks through the top of the lens where optics are more stable for distance vision at any distant object and check the clarity of vision as shown in the Figure 11.21.

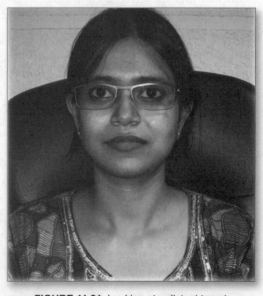

FIGURE 11.21: Looking at a distant target

2. Demonstrate the near vision—ask him to hold a reading card at his habitual distance and check the clarity of vision. In order to do so instruct the wearer to slowly lift his chin while continuing to look at the stationary near target to find whether the near target appears clear as shown in Figure 11.22.

3. Now demonstrate the blurriness from top to bottom of the lens—ask the wearer to fixate at the distant object again and then gradually lift the chin so that the middle and lower portions of the lens are used and let him feel the increasing blurriness.

4. Demonstrating the mid-distance vision—ask the patient to extend his hand as shown in Figure 11.23 and slowly raise the gaze to look through the mid-portion of the lens.

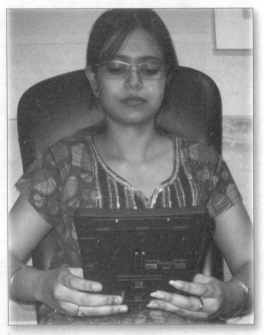

FIGURE 11.22: Chin up and gaze down to look at reading object

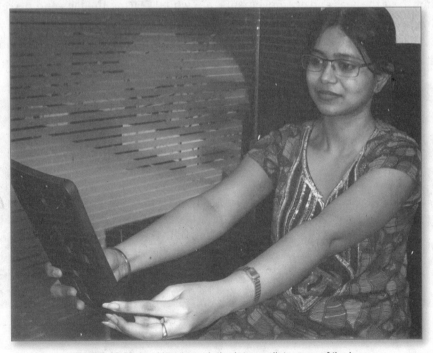

FIGURE 11.23: Looking through the Intermediate zone of the lens

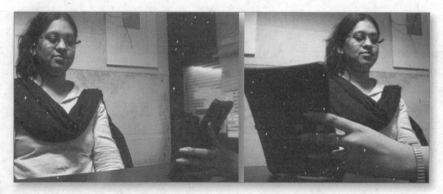

FIGURE 11.24: Demonstrating the vision at various angles of gazes

5. Demonstrating the vision at various angles of gazes—while the wearer holds a reading card, place the objects at different intermediate distances on both sides of dispensing table and in front of the patient as shown in Figure 11.24. And let him feel how side vision affects the clarity.

6. Demonstrate the head and eye movement during lateral gaze—only eye movement is the incorrect way of using progressive addition lens. Once the eyes are turned, head posture is adjusted to use the lens effectively as shown in Figure 11.25.

7. Demonstrate eye movement on staircase —while going up or down on the staircase look through the mid-portion of the lens as shown in Figure 11.26.

8. Demonstrate the mobility with the lens—ask him to walk around the office while wearing the lens and perceive any blur or waviness in the periphery. If the wearer notices mild blur or waviness, he is likely to adapt.

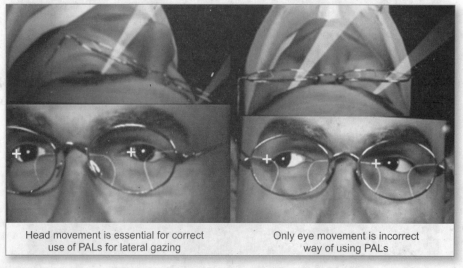

Head movement is essential for correct use of PALs for lateral gazing

Only eye movement is incorrect way of using PALs

FIGURE 11.25: Demonstrating head and eye movement while using progressive addition lens

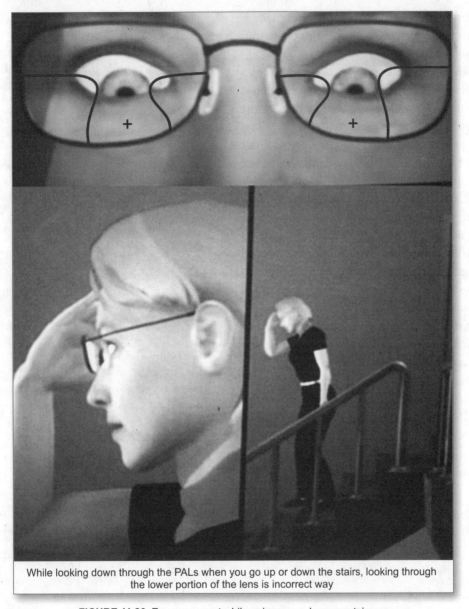

While looking down through the PALs when you go up or down the stairs, looking through the lower portion of the lens is incorrect way

FIGURE 11.26: Eye movement while going up or down on staircase

The total demonstration gives the wearer a fair deal of idea about how the lenses need to be used for various distances and makes the adaptation easier and smoother. However, a word of caution that the wearer must learn to depress his eyes by larger amount than for segmented bifocal lenses to be really successful with progressive lenses. Some wearer also finds it difficult to locate the right zone to look through. Since progressives lenses have no lines, it does not clearly identify the various viewing zones; hence clarity is the only reference for them to understand the position of various viewing zones.

The overall success in progressive lens dispensing needs an in depth knowledge about the lenses because there will be some cases where the patient will fail to adapt to progressive lenses. The possibilities can be minimized by prudently selecting an appropriate candidate for progressive addition lens. Patients who are prone to vertigo, who work on heights, or those who are not ready to accept changes may be avoided. An in depth thoughts are needed before prescribing progressive lenses to anisometropes or patients with high oblique astigmatisms. Besides, care should be taken to avoid dispensing half pair progressive lenses. Prism thinning that produces vertical prisms may differ and ultimately may produce unwanted prismatic effect. Prism thinning is incorporated to equalize the thickness at the top and bottom edge of the progressive lenses. The amount of prism thinning applied to a lens is dependent on the add power.

POINTS TO REMEMBER

- 2 small hidden engraving are permanently etched at 17 mm on either side of the PRP, i.e. they are 34 mm apart on the horizontal line.
- Temporary ink marking are very important for lens dispensing and are always utilized to position the lens during lens glazing, lens fitting and verifications.
- The distance reference point (DRP) represents the location on the surface that provides the exact base curve and is the optimal location for verifying the distance prescription.
- The near reference point (NRP) represents the location on the surface that provides full target near addition and is surrounded by the near power circle.
- The length of the progressive corridor is usually defined as the distance from the fitting cross to the top edge of the stable near power circle.
- The longer corridor progressive requires more eye depression at the reading position.
- Patient must learn to depress the eyes by larger amount than the segmented multifocal lenses to really appreciate the progressive lens benefits.
- The PRP in PAL is located at the GC of the lens.
- Prism is measured at the midway between the horizontal alignment engravings, i.e. at PRP or GC or DOC.
- As the add power of a progressive lens increases, the unwanted cylinder power typically increases.

PRISM DISPENSING

Prismatic corrections are prescribed when there is failure of both eyes to direct their gaze simultaneously at the same object in space due to imbalance of the extraocular muscles to achieve one fused image or in other words when eye muscles do not move together in harmony. Whenever prisms are prescribed, it entails certain unique considerations to dispense, because any amount of error may cause visual problems for patients including blur, headaches, nausea and even double vision. Chapter 12 explains dispensing issues related to prism dispensing.

A prism is a triangular piece of transparent material whose refracting surfaces are inclined at an angle to each other to intersect at apex. The side opposite to apex is known as base of the prism. In practice, thinner portion is known as apex and thicker portion is known as base of the prism. The rays of light passing through the prism will bend towards the base of the prism and the image would appear to shift towards the apex of the prism. However, prism does not cause any change in vergence of light. In ophthalmic optics prisms are usually used for correction of symptomatic binocular vision disorders.

Prisms are usually prescribed with reference to the orientation of their base as base out, base in, base up and base down when the directions are horizontal and vertical as shown in the Figures 12.1 and 12.2. In all other base directions require 360° notation of compass. For example, RE 2▲ at 160° as shown in Figure 12.3.

When the prisms are prescribed in the prescription by an eyecare practitioner, the optician needs to incorporate the prescribed prism in the ophthalmic lenses. The optical effects of the prism are noticed as under:

- Prism on eyes causes eye to move towards the apex of the prism. When base out prism is placed in front of an eye, the eye moves inwards and when base in prism is placed in front of an

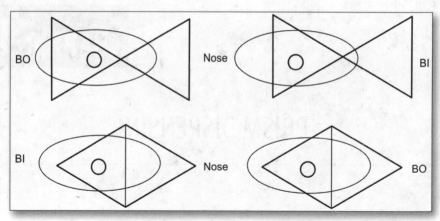

FIGURE 12.1: Orientation of horizontal prisms

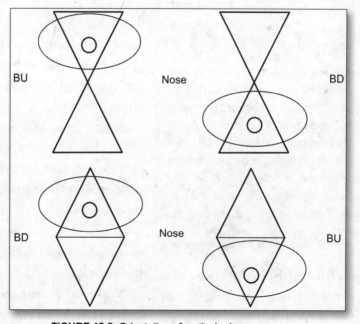

FIGURE 12.2: Orientation of vertical prisms

eye, the eye moves outwards as shown in Figure 12.4.

- Prism in ophthalmic lens causes shifting of optical center of the lens. The optical center of the lens shifts towards base of the prism in plus power and it shifts towards the apex of the prism minus power.

- When base in prism is used on eyes, it minimizes the need for convergence. Therefore, it is good for a patient having exophoria.

- When base out prism is used on eyes, it increases the need for convergence. Therefore, it is good for a patient having esophoria.

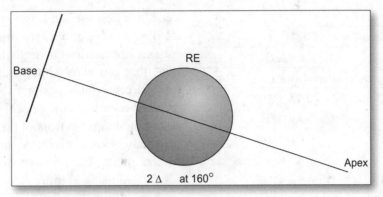

FIGURE 12.3: Orientation of prism in right eye

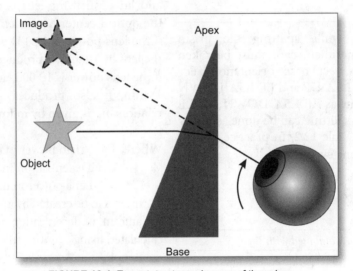

FIGURE 12.4: Eye rotates towards apex of the prism

- Vertical prisms are very critical, even the smaller amount of vertical prism may produce symptoms.
- Prism in lens blurs vision.

Thus, prisms alleviate symptoms associated with disorder of binocular vision by deviating light to fall on the foveae of both eyes.

The prescribed prism is usually divided equally between the two eyes to:

- Distribute the weight more evenly
- Reduce thickness of the intended lens
- Minimize chromatic aberration
- Minimize the effect of reduction in blur.

For example, right eye 3▲ IN causes right eye to deviate outwards by 3▲. If we place 1.5▲ IN before each eye, the required total deviation will be still achieved. Therefore, RE 3▲ IN can be divided as RE 1.5▲ IN combined with LE 1.5▲ IN. Such a division in the horizontal meridian does not have to be equal in magnitude. An example is given in Table 12.1 for 4 prism base out.

Table 12.1:

Splitting 4 prism base out in two eyes	
RE Zero	LE 4▲ OUT
R combined with L	
0.5▲ OUT	3.5▲ OUT
1▲ OUT	3▲ OUT
1.5▲ OUT	2.5▲ OUT
2▲ OUT	2▲ OUT
2.5▲ OUT	1.5▲ OUT
3▲ OUT	1▲ OUT
3.5▲ OUT	0.5▲ OUT
4▲ OUT	Zero

However, while splitting the prism in vertical meridian, care must be taken to ensure correct base orientation. For example, RE 1.5▲ UP and LE 1.5▲ DOWN is not the same as RE 1.5▲ DOWN and LE 1.5▲UP. The splitting can be done as under as shown in Table 12.2. In practice usually splitting is done evenly.

Table 12.2:

Splitting vertical prism	
RE 3▲ UP	LE Zero
R combined with L	
0.5▲ UP	2.5▲ DOWN
1▲ UP	2▲ DOWN
1.5▲ UP	1.5▲ DOWN
2▲ UP	1▲ DOWN
2.5▲ UP	0.5▲ DOWN
3▲ UP	Zero

There are 2 ways of incorporating the prescribed prism—either it can be created by lens decentration or prisms can be worked during lens surfacing.

PRISM BY DECENTRATION

Prism by decentration is the simplest method to incorporate the prism in the spectacle lens. It is best used in lenses with moderate to high powers, and where small amount of prisms are needed. It needs a large uncut lens that can allow shifting or placing the optical center at a position desired by the prescribed prism. The optical center of the lens is no longer in front of the pupil, hence prismatic effect is created at the optical center point. The required decentration is calculated using Prentice rule. Prentice rule says that there is a relationship between the magnitude of prism, the power of the lens, and how much the lens is decenterd from the optical center of the lens. For example, if the lens power is 1.00 D and we decenter the lens by 10 mm, it produces 1D prism. Or if the lens power is 10.00 D and we decenter 1 mm, it also produces 1D prism. The relationship is given by following equation:

$P = cF$

Where, P = Prism power in diopter

c = Decentration in centimeter

F = Lens power in diopter

If 1Δ is to be created by a −1.00 Dsph lens, the amount of decentration needed would be calculated using Prentice rule as under:

$P = cF$

$1Δ = c × 1$

$1/1 = c$

$c = 1$ cm

So the lens must be decentered by 1 cm or 10 mm.

The sequential process of creating prism by decentration is as follows:

1. Use the Prentice rule to calculate the decentration required.
2. Put the mark on the demo lens where IPD would be positioned after decentration.
3. Calculate the uncut size lens needed for the frame by calculating effective diameter.

4. Lens is glazed so as to fit the optical center at the marked place of the demo lens.

It is also not possible to create prism by decentration in case of aspheric lens, as this will alter the optics of the lens.

WORKED PRISMS

When the prescribed prism is higher or the lens diameter falls short of required decentration, prism has to be worked on the lenses during lens surfacing. The worked prism is created by creating the edge thickness difference of the uncut lens; and thereby effecting the shifting of the optical center position of the lens. During lens surfacing the thickness at the apex and the thickness at the base is controlled over a specific diameter as calculated by the require decentration. It works exactly in the same way. The required prism diopter is calculated using the following equation:

$$d = 10 \times P / D$$
$$P = D \times d / 10$$

where, d = Decentration in millimeter

D = Diopter or lens power

P = Prism degree

Then it is ground by keeping the edge difference for which the equation is:

Edge difference = Prism × size of lens × 0.019.

The process of creating worked prism as under:

1. Use the above equation to calculate the prism diopter needed for required decentration.
2. Calculate the required edge difference needed using edge difference equation.

3. Measure the patient's IPD and put the mark on the demo lens where IPD would be positioned.
4. Lens is glazed so as to fit the geometrical center of the lens at the marked place on the demo lens.

COMPOUND AND RESOLVING PRISMS

Prisms may be prescribed by specifying the amount of prism together with its direction of orientation using 360° notation of compass. This is quite common for oblique and compounded prisms; 0 is always positioned right on the lens and 180 on left, and 90 superiorly and 270 inferiorly. For example, a given prescription calls for a vertical prism in conjunction with a horizontal prism in left eye as

LE 3▲ BD with 4▲ BO

The combined effect of above prism could be produced by a single prism of appropriate power with its base in some oblique setting.

To find the single prism, draw an accurate diagram. Remember standard notations, which say that the axis starts at 0 on the right hand side of each eye and goes around anticlockwise from the observer's point of view as shown in Figure 12.5.

Draw a set of lines at right angles to one another and mark the nasal area along with the primary directions based on this as shown in Figure 12.6.

Picking a suitable scale, i.e. 1 cm = 1 diopter, mark a point equivalent to 3▲ down and 4▲ out as shown in Figure 12.7.

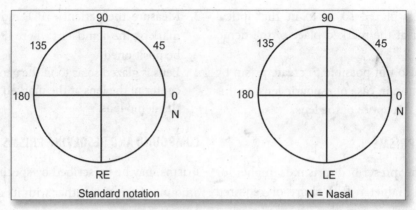

FIGURE 12.5: 360 notations on compass

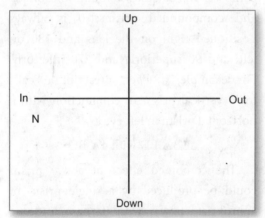

FIGURE 12.6: Left eye representation showing principal direction

Now construct a rectangle based on this and draw in a diagonal from the center of the cross lines to the corner of the rectangle as drawn in Figure 12.8.

This line represents both the magnitude and the base setting of the resultant prism. The line measures 5 units and therefore equals 5▲ diopters. The direction in relation to the center of the cross lines and nasal area is down and out. Expressed in terms of a 360° notation the base direction is 323°.

If a 180° notation is required the diagonal line needs to be extended so that it lies above

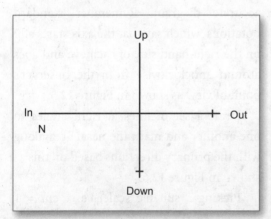

FIGURE 12.7: Shows 3 base down and 4 base out to scale

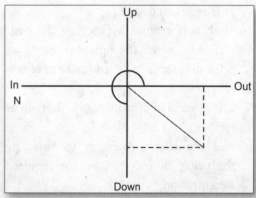

FIGURE 12.8: Construction completed to show magnitude and angle of oblique prism

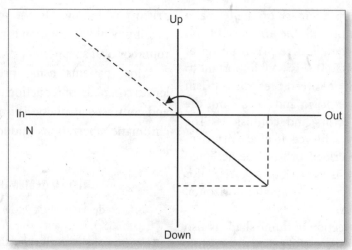

Up

In ——————————————— Out

N

Down

FIGURE 12.9: Showing angle of prism in standard notation

the horizontal, measuring the axis indicated as shown in Figure 12.9. Therefore, the answer to compounding the prisms is:

5▲ base at 143° out

or, 5▲ base at 323°

There is a mathematical solution to compounding prisms. The formula is:

$$P_R = \sqrt{P_V^2 + P_H^2}$$

where,

P_R = Single resultant prism

P_V = Prism vertical

P_H = Prism horizontal

Putting the values from the previous example—

$$P_R = \sqrt{3^2 + 4^2}$$
$$P_R = \sqrt{9 + 16}$$
$$P_R = \sqrt{25}$$
$$P_R = 5▲$$

Now to obtain the base setting use:

$$\tan \Theta = \frac{P_V}{P_H}$$
$$\tan \Theta = ¾$$
$$\tan \Theta = 37°$$

This needs to be converted to standard notation by subtracting from 180° (180–37= 143)

Therefore, the answer is 143°.

CHALLENGES ASSOCIATED WITH PRISM DISPENSING

When prisms are prescribed there is a displacement of the visual world to which the wearer has to adapt. Adaptation depends on the interaction between the motor and the sensory systems that occurs in brain. Image senses through the eyes are relayed to the visual cortex of the brain where the brain accounts for the difference and allows the patient to perceive the world as "normal." Adaptation is subjective. Some patients adapt quickly and some takes little longer time. There are some who fail to adapt. One of the most important factors that determine the success while dispensing prism is effective prism has to be same as prescribed prism. Correct placement of prism is really a challenging job. Before measuring the prism power in the lens, it is important to put a mark on the lens at a point that lines up with the line of sight and then measure the effective prism power at the marked point. This is very important to ensure similarity between prescribed prism and the effective prism and to rule out the possibility of errors and confusions. The success is only achieved if effective prism equals the prescribed prism. The accepted tolerance limit as prescribed by ANSI for vertical prism is ±0.33 Δ and for horizontal prism is ±0.67 Δ.

The ideal selection of frame shape is also very critical for successful prism dispensing. Square or rectangular shapes with sharp corners do not allow lenses to rotate while the lens is fitted and thus ensure stable prism positioning. On the other hand the possibility of lens rotation is more in case of round or oval shape frames.

Most patients using prism corrected lenses complain of reduction in visual acuity and contrast sensitivity. This may be due to chromatic aberrations induced by prism lenses.

POINT TO REMEMBER

- Prism deviates light towards its base without changing its vergence.
- Prisms are prescribed with reference to their base orientation.
- Prisms may be divided in two eyes equally or unequally.

CHAPTER 13

DISPENSING PRESCRIPTION SUNGLASSES

Sunglasses are healthcare products that also add an extra "zing" to the appearance of the wearer. Prescription sunglasses improve visual performance and can also be used as ocular defense gadget. While selecting a suitable sunglass you need to make sure that the sunglasses fit your face properly and serve its desired purpose. The objective of Chapter 13 is to acquaint the reader with challenges associated with prescription sunglass dispensing.

Good looks are the snare that everybody would like to be caught in. Most people buy their sunglasses as a fashion accessory. They need to understand that sunglasses are not just the fashion accessory; they are also a healthcare need that also serves occupational and functional needs. Modern sunglasses are real technologically driven products. A good quality sunglass is made with highly sophisticated technology and before it reaches to the wearer it passes through lot of stringent quality control tests. Each sunglass is tested for:

1. Impact resistance

2. Light absorption and transmission
3. Glare control
4. Reflection prevention
5. Surface regularity
6. Nonionizing radiation protection.

They are designed to achieve not only cosmetic objectives but also healthcare objectives to:

1. Protect eyes from light, heat and trauma.
2. Enhance contrast.
3. Prevent ocular fatigue.
4. Prevent color distortion.
5. Improve visual performance.
6. Minimize any disadvantages.
7. And above all to prevent all those factors that take a toll on the eyes and brain.

Spending too much time outdoors in the summer sun may raise the risk of a common sight-robbing disease later in the life. There are immediate effects also. Too much of light causes glare. Glare is a condition in which it is difficult to keep the eyes open. Squinting of eyes is one of the most commonly seen activities among the people in order to prevent the effect of glare. Some people also shield their eyes using their hands or assume typical look of contempt in order to prevent eyes from glare. It also impairs visual performance and results in various other symptoms. It has been proved that long-term exposures of the eyes to nonradiation have aging effect, specially in the form of early macular degeneration and cataract. Besides, there are other damaging effects noticed in the form of pinguecula and pterygium. Those who spend most of their time near rivers, ocean and mountains are more susceptible to sunlight. People of all ages should take precautions whenever they are outdoors. It is, therefore recommended to use UV absorbent sunglasses and a brimmed hat whenever a person is in the sun for long periods of time. The use of sunglasses is particularly indicated in the following circumstances:

- During the summer when sun shine is at its peak the level of UV radiation is increased.
- While on sea beach.
- On high altitudes while participating in winter sports.
- Some medications may can cause light sensitivity, using sunglasses may help while you are on those medication.
- Those who develop ocular media opacity will tend to become more sensitive to light because of the light scattering effect, even if they were not naturally light sensitive.

TINTS FOR SUNGLASSES

The different wavelengths of light across visible spectrum give rise to different color sensation. Based upon their wavelength values they provide different advantages to the wearer. Violet, blue and indigo are at the shorter wavelength end of the visible light.

They may carry enormous amount of UV rays together with them. They also focus in front of retina, creating light scattering effect within the globe. Hence they may not be considered good for outdoor use specially when the light is poor. While prescribing blue tint for outdoor use, it would be prudent to prescribe either greenish-blue or grayish-blue tint which would absorb the UV rays. Green has very good UV and IR absorption properties. It also absorbs shorter wavelengths of blue light and lies around the peak of spectral acuity at 500 nm. It implies that it transmits more light and thus enhances visual information and it also has good heat absorption properties. That is why it is more natural choice of people who are light sensitive with a preference of quieter color. Yellow lies at the peak spectral acuity and anyone who is particularly light sensitive will have aversion to yellow tint. Orange and red lie near the longer wavelength end of the visible light. They absorb UV and blue and therefore enhance contrast, but they also carry thermal effect of infrared rays with them. They are mostly used for sunglass purpose by minimizing their intensity of spectral color and alter its perception considerably with low intensity orange-yellow with black that results in brown tint. Brown tint provides good contrast and at the same time prevents UV transmission. Another very popular tint for sunglasses is gray which is a neutral density filter. It is good for light sensitive people and also for jobs which requires accurate color discrimination. In fact the choice of gray tint for sunglass use is most natural. Tints may be of different types, common among them are:

1. Solid tints
2. Gradient tints
3. Mirror coated
4. Polaroid.

Solid Tints

Resin lenses can be fully tinted by immersing in a container of dye. The container is put in a unit that allows heat to be transferred to the dye. The longer the lenses remain in the dye, the more dye will be absorbed and the lens will be darker. The dye penetrates the lens material and becomes the part of it.

Gradient Tints

Graduated tints are darker at the top of the lens and gradually become lighter as you go towards the bottom of the lens. The graduated effects are comparatively easy to achieve with the aid of a pulley mechanism which gradually lifts the lenses out of the tint tank, thus imparting more tint on one part of the lens than the other. They are good tint of choice for prescription sunglasses with presbyopic correction as light bottom portion of the lens facilitates reading.

Mirror Coated Lenses

A mirror coating can be applied by a vacuum process to the front surface of the lens causing the lens to have the same properties as a two way mirror. Mirror coatings are often used in combination with a tinted lens to provide more protection from intense sunlight. Mirror coated lenses work by reflecting back specific wavelengths, whereas solid tints work by absorbing the wavelengths or light energy. Light energy so absorbed expresses itself in the form of heat which might irradiate the eyes. But this does not occur in case of vacuum tints as the energy is reflected away.

Polaroid Lenses

The world is full of glare. The only way to counteract the nature's glare is to use polarized sunglasses. Polaroid lenses are dispensed to protect the eyes from the ill-effect of horizontal waves that cause glare and reduce the visual performance. Rays of light that are reflected by surface materials travels horizontally and together with the incident light waves creates light pollution. The overall visual effect of light pollution is glare and loss of contrast. Polarized lenses can be useful in controlling the transmission of horizontal light waves since they have the property of filtering out reflected light. This is being made possible by inclusion of some crystals, such as quartz, tourmaline and calcite that can suppress the light vibration in a particular direction. Polaroid lenses are good for water and snow sports people, but are contraindicated for people working with LCD display. While fitting into the frame, care must be taken to fit the lenses keeping the microetching horizontally.

LENS MATERIAL FOR SUNGLASSES

Sunglasses are also used as safety lenses. Together with other safety devices, polycarbonate lens material is important defense gadget for athletes and all those who are engaged in fast occupation used for ocular protection. Polycarbonate is roughly 10 times impact-resistant than CR 39 lens material. They make the lenses to work like a shield lenses to protect the eyes from traumatic blows. It has an added advantage of being very light in weight with high refractive index. The material also has built in UV protection advantage. However, the material is softer which makes it more prone to scratches. The lenses are, therefore, made with scratch-resistant coating. Trivex is another lens material that can be ideally used for sunglasses. Like polycarbonate lens material, lenses made of Trivex are thinner, lighter and more impact-resistant than regular plastic or glass lenses. Trivex has a slightly lower refractive index (1.53 compared to 1.58), its specific gravity, 1.11g/cm³, makes it the lightest of any lens material available today. Like polycarbonate, Trivex also has inbuilt UV protection. However, unlike polycarbonate, Trivex has an Abbe value of 45, making it optically superior to polycarbonate lens material.

LENS DESIGN FOR SUNGLASSES

Aspheric lens design is most ideally suited lens design for prescription sunglasses as they enhance the cosmetic appearance of the sunglasses and also enhance the peripheral awareness. Flatter lens also reduces the lens mass, making the lens lighter in weight. Weight is very important factor for stability specially in fast and vigorous activities. However, lenses need to be customized to match the wrap curve of the sports sunglasses. Sports frame differs with conventional dress wear frame in terms of fitting on the face. High-curve lenses are needed to fit the lenses into sports frames. Until recently, lenses for sports frames have been made by producing the patient's prescription using high spherical base lenses which typically had a nominal front curve of 8.25 D or 9.25 D. It implies that the rule of "best form lenses" is not followed. The results have been noticed as unwanted prisms, radial astigmatism and

blur vision that adversely affects the lens for central and peripheral power. New sports lenses are designed to compensate for these unwanted errors and to provide desired visual performance through the lens central and peripheral portion. Although they differ in lens power when verified with lens prescription, they do provide desired subjective responses. This has been made possible because of three-dimensional optical correction, not just two-dimensional used for conventional lenses. Sports is a high speed activity in which our eyes work like a multitask performer. There is no room for any compromise in the visual performance in sports. Specially designed sports lenses with surface treatments work wonderfully to increase central and peripheral visual performance through the lenses.

ANTIREFLECTION COATING FOR SUNGLASSES

There is no doubt that dispensing of antireflection (AR) coatings in general is on steep slope of growth. A major thrust is applying AR coatings on all lenses. Adding a premium coating to a premium lens seems to agree with consumers also. One of the most important advantages that antireflection coated lenses provides is the increase in light transmittance through the lenses, which means even with dark tints the wearer can enjoy increased visual performance. In addition, reduction of reflections off the backside of the lens also enhances vision and comfort. Sun lenses with a frontside AR coating can enhance the wearer's appearance by reducing distracting reflections off the front of the lens. However, there is some debate on whether to coat frontside and/or backside sun lenses. Back surface reflection is the common problem of sun lenses, i.e. the light that hits the back of the lenses and bounces into the eyes. In bad cases, you can actually see the reflection of your eye in the lens. The purpose of an AR coating is to reduce these reflections off the lenses. Sometimes AR coatings are also applied to the front of prescription sunglasses to eliminate the "hot spot" glare that reflects off the lens. However, with the very dark lenses, you do not really get the glare on the frontside, and if you do coat it, you can get a rainbow look to the dark lens. Polarized lenses are coated only at their backside because coating on the front surface may reduces the effect of the polarization and coating on the back of polarized lens means you do not even have to fight little reflections that annoy your eyes.

New researches are aiming to justify the need of sunglasses to prevent the effect of jetlag, improve reading performances and reduce the effect of migraines. Specially designed sunglasses are needed in space too, where sunlight is far more intense and harmful than on the Earth. Lifestyle sunglasses are integral part of total accessories. They are the most observed and noticed among all. In fact you are not complete without a good sunglass on your eyes. Not to forget they also enhance contact lens wearing comfort. Use of sunglass in daylight may help improve your dark adaptation. Vision is the function of contrast sensitivity. A correct filter selected for your sunglasses will also have a long term effect on the preservation of visual acuity.

POINTS TO REMEMBER

- Over exposure to nonionizing radiations contributes to an aging effect in our eyes.
- Green tint has very good UV and IR absorption properties.
- Mirror coated lenses work by reflecting back specific wavelengths, whereas solid tints work by absorbing the wavelengths or light energy.
- Polaroid lenses are dispensed to protect the eyes from the ill-effect of horizontal waves that cause glare and reduce the visual performance.
- A polarizing lens should be oriented so as to eliminate horizontally vibrating waves
- Polycarbonate is roughly 10 times impact resistant than CR 39 lens material.
- Antireflection coating on the back of polarized lens means you do not even have to fight little reflections that annoy your eyes.

OCCUPATIONAL DISPENSING OF SPECTACLE

Today optical dispensing is seen as an important part of holistic eye care that goes beyond the normal scope to include preventions and enhancements. A person may not show competent occupational performance due to a disruption in his visual ability that is limited by the correction modality. Dysfunction occurs because the person's ability to adapt has been challenged to the point that the demands for performance are not satisfactorily met. Chapter 14 aims to explain how occupational performance can be improved by applying the concept of occupational dispensing.

The history of human civilization reflects a progressive change in the human culture and their behavior. From hunting to the current technological era, it has passed through dramatic evolutionary changes. The dynamism of evolutionary developments has brought various changes in the behavior pattern of the human being. Hunters of past are now confined to four walls of offices and houses. The result is our entire viewing world is now restricted to boundaries of those walls. This has changed our visual demands from more of distance vision to more of near vision. The predominance of "near point world" implies that the eyes are in a constant state of accommodation creating a sustained stress on visual system. Moreover, the increased complexities of various occupations have added fuel to it. Occupations are everything we do in our life. In other words, occupations explain how we relate to our environment. These occupations include activities that consist of 3 important properties as shown in the Flowchart 14.1.

All the occupational interactions may be summarized as behavior. Vision and visual responses are one such behavior. 90% of the interaction with the environment is through the vision. Each occupational interaction creates unique visual demands that ask the person concerned to respond in unique way. Any deficiency in vision and visual system may influence the interaction adversely and thereby affect occupational performance. However, nature has designed our visual system to be so dominant that we adapt our visual system to accommodate

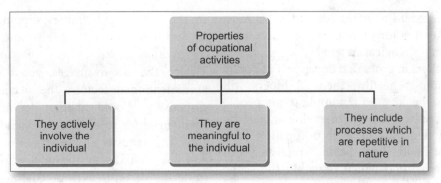

FLOWCHART 14.1: 3 important properties of occupational activities

any deficiency in the way we see. In the process we overlook other bodily function ability and tend to assume typical postures. For high visually demanding task, the effect is on the entire body that creates additional stress on muscles. This happens when the visual response does not meet the challenges of the occupation and visual demands exceed the visual abilities, the individual has to modify or adjust his behavior to achieve the required competence. The effect is seen on overall occupational performance leading to dissatisfaction and frustrations. Earlier the clinical justification of the optometric practice has been known in terms of the detection of deficiency and their management. The preventive and enhancement side of the optometry have been very much underestimated which also falls within the realm of dispensing optics and is conceptualized as occupational dispensing. Today the dispensing of spectacle is being seen as an important part of holistic eye care that goes beyond the normal scope to include prevention and enhancements. The dispensing opticians look at an individual patient, analyze his visual needs and accordingly provide the solution to maintain required competence in their occupation. Thus occupational dispensing is an important part of holistic eye care. The dispensing optician considers several components of occupational dispensing before designing a suitable solution. The important components are shown in the Flowchart 14.2.

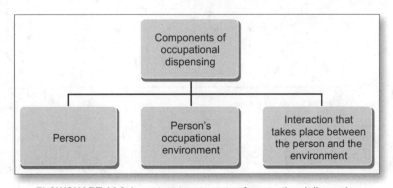

FLOWCHART 14.2: Important components of occupational dispensing

The extension of the concept is that most people often forget that eyes are the part of same physiological system as the legs, hands and others in general. If one aspect of bodily function is healthy, then all others will also be healthy. So in simple terms people who really wants to meet the increasing visual demands of their occupation have to work with their specific visual needs of the occupation which is within the scope of dispensing optics. It is, therefore the professional responsibility of the dispensing optician to take care of visual behavior of the individual with respect to the visual demands of the occupation to achieve the desired objectives as shown in Flowchart 14.3.

Vision Enhancement

The primary aim of occupational dispensing is to enhance the visual performance for the specific occupation. The visual demands of the occupation are analyzed and suitable corrections are designed to enhance the visual performance with an aim to enhance the occupational performance.

Minimize Disadvantage

Occupational environment, compromised correction for the working distance, glare in the visual field, frames slipping, poor fit and steaming up are also the reason for compromised visual performance. Where the disadvantages occur due to aforementioned factors, the occupational dispensing should attempt to minimize them in order to elevate the standards of care. This requires all the arts of refraction and the best dispensing advice available, in terms of antireflection coating, tinted lenses, scratch resistance lenses, anti-mist and water repellent coating to maximize contrast, reduce glare and minimize any disadvantage.

Protection from Trauma and Radiation

Protection in addition to vision is another function of the eyewear. The main sources of traumatic injury come from a direct blow to the eye or the adnexa and nonionizing radiations. The use of shatter proof lens material, UV rays protection lenses and other specially designed appliances are available to protect against these sources of trauma and radiations.

Example

- *Person*: A young 30-year-old male with versatile and fast lifestyle.

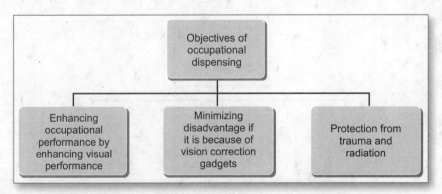

FLOWCHART 14.3: 3 important objectives of occupational dispensing

- *Occupational environment*: Drives a lot and primarily outdoor job.
- *Visual interaction*: The person needs to visit construction sites at various locations where his occupational visual demands are inspections of sites and work in progress, primarily engaged in distance ·and near viewing tasks in outdoor environment.
- *Vision enhancement*: Prescription sunglass with brown tint facilitates driving by ensuring glare protection and contrast enhancement during noon and evening hours.
- *Minimize disadvantage*: Prescription sunglass lenses can be treated with back surface antireflection coating to minimize the effect of reflection from lens back surface for driving and site inspection.
- *Protection*: Sunglasses can be dispensed in polycarbonate lenses to ensure protection from UV and dust particles, stones and other missiles that may be lead to traumatic injury.
- *Proposed solution*: A prescription sunglass dispensed with polycarbonate lens with back surface antireflection coating will help enhance his occupational work and a general purpose antireflection lenses with clear tint will help indoor or dim light occupational activities. The proposed solution will not only enhance vision but also protect and maintain vision to ensure the holistic eye care.

3 SIMPLE RULES

The concept of occupational dispensing is based on the assumption that people have inherent drive for mastery and in order to achieve mastery in their occupations they are ready to undergo an experimental process that allow them to try new and modern tools and gadgets to enhance their occupational performance. The straight forward meaning is there is a scope where an optician can get into the occupational needs of the person and apply the concept of occupational dispensing successfully. 3 simple rules as shown in the Flowchart 14.4 facilitate the practice to apply the art of occupational dispensing.

1. Asking questions are the simplest way to apply occupational dispensing. If you do not know the visual demand of a person, you cannot provide the solution and the only way to know the visual demand is putting up interrogative type questions. Questions pertaining to type of work, hobbies, activities done for recreation and any specific visual needs may give optician comprehensive information about the visual demands of a person.

2. Once you know the visual needs, you need to restate and express your concern as to disadvantages that are being associated with current mode of correction modality or stresses involved in the occupations because not many people have any idea about what they are missing by not using a desired solution.

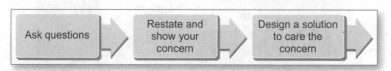

FLOWCHART 14.4: 3 simple rules to practice occupational dispensing

3. Once the patient understands, he will be looking at the optician for solution. It is the responsibility of the optician to provide suitable solution. Solutions may be prescribed from amongst the list of occupational specific gadgets available or a specific modality may be designed for him. While providing the solution the optician must explain the benefits and advantage of the prescribed solution—what he will be gaining if he uses and what he will be missing if he does not use.

OCCUPATIONAL SPECIFIC GADGETS

A number of frames and lenses have been designed as occupation specific gadgets. Broadly speaking their fitting procedure is based on the same principles as that of traditional spectacles. The difference lies in the unique consideration needed to dispense them.

Billiards Spectacle

Spectacle frames incorporating joints at or below the datum line which enables the wearer to see through the top portion of the lens in a leaning down position are popularly used as billiards or snooker spectacles as shown in Figure 14.1. They facilitate visual performance while playing snooker or billiards.

Clip On

Clip ons are attachments to provide an additional lens which may be used as sunglass or add on power. They are fitted in front of spectacle frame by means of hooks or spring action as shown in Figure 14.2.

Flip Up Frames

There are several variants that have one thing in common; the frames are fitted with a secondary front that can be swiveled upwards as shown in Figure 14.3. The secondary front may be used to fit protective lenses or near or distance vision lenses.

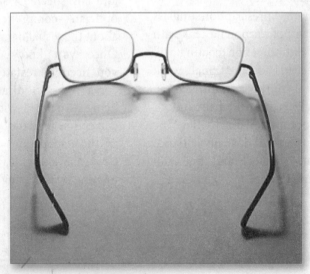

FIGURE 14.1: Billiards spectacle

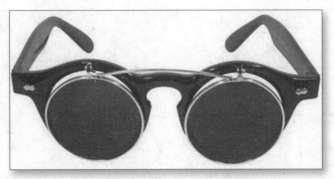

FIGURE 14.2: Clip on spectacle

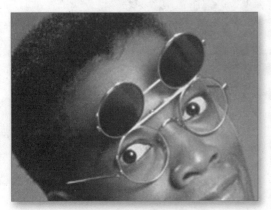

FIGURE 14.3: Flip up frame

Flying Frames (Fig. 14.4)

Large sizes in pilot-shaped goggles allow obtaining view as high and wide as possible. However, this adds to the weight and to peripheral distortion. Loop end sides and brow bar help to stabilize frames. Spectacle frame sides should neither interfere with a radio headset nor should be uncomfortable during wear.

Half Eye Spectacle

Half eye reading spectacles are very good

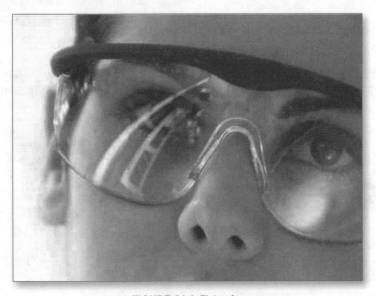

FIGURE 14.4: Flying frames

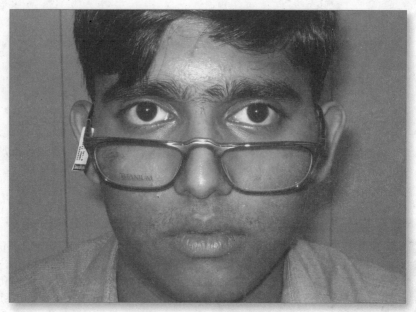

FIGURE 14.5: Half eye spectacle

option for reading in supine position or for prolonged reading job. Reading half eye spectacles as shown in Figure 14.5 can be suggested together with regular pair to read while sleeping or for longer reading hours.

Industrial Protection Spectacle

The British and European Standards for eye protectors, USA .... ANSI Z 87.1, Canada .... CSA Z 94, etc. are various standards that describe the basic requirements and basic designs for industrial protection spectacles. Some of the common features are width of the frames is larger, nosepiece is softer, overall weight is lighter, temples are flexible and are made of tough materials like polycarbonate as shown in Figure 14.6.

Swimming Goggles

Swimming goggles are designed with individual cup type lenses incorporating an

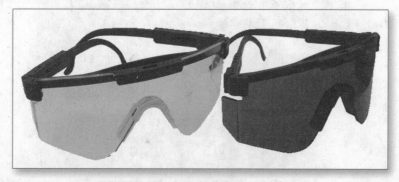

FIGURE 14.6: Industrial protection spectacle

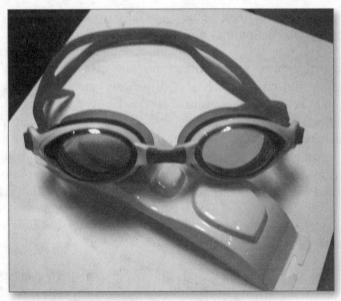

FIGURE 14.7: Swimming glasses

eye seal as shown in Figure 14.7. They are used for surface swimming only.

Sports Frames

Sports frames are designed to follow the contours of the face. The wrap shape frames have larger "A" measurement than "B" measurement and fits closer to the eyes. Some sports frames have strap which passes behind the head, instead of conventional sides.

Enhanced Near Vision Lenses

These lenses are so designed that the upper portion of the lens is used to see at an intermediate distance and the bottom portion is used for near work. It is very good option for presbyope who is an avid user of computer, pilots, surgeons and many others. Avid card player would enjoy wide intermediate and larger near-extended near vision lenses.

Anti-Fatigue Lenses

Anti-fatigue lenses are designed for younger people who spend lot of their time on computer, electronic games and other near work which requires increased attention. The lenses support the wearer accommodative efforts while working at shorter distance.

The concept behind occupational dispensing is to address the patient's specific vocational visual needs. Considerations should be given to patient's needs, discussion of available options, how they will help remediate the concern and follow ups. The specific lens may not be a very complicated one. Idea is to reinforce the fact that one pair of lenses possibly will not meet all the visual demands a person has right from the morning to night. Sometimes a correct selection of tint can make a difference. Lot more can be explored, in fact the optician needs to have small brain storming session before devising a suitable solution. Some of the following simplest solution may also work:

- A presbyopic patient who works with electronics using mid-range vision all the day—a good choice is single vision intermediate powered lens designed for his working distance.
- Prescription sunglasses can be recommended for a person who works or plays outside. Poloroid lenses are very good.
- Anti-fog treated lenses can be dispensed to prevent the lens fogging in the air-condition car.
- A segmented bifocal lens may be prescribed for intermediate and near vision.
- Polycarbonate lenses may be used for safety purpose. Power sunglasses can be made for outdoor use.
- Daily disposable soft contact lenses may be used for surface swimming.
- An additional amber tint with ARC coating may be used for night driving.
- Oblong shape lenses with holes drilled around the datum line can be designed in a rimless frame for billiards player.

The key to success lies in explaining the patient that the occupational lenses are special purpose lenses and not for general use. Using them for other than intended purpose is absolutely contraindicated and may not yield good results. Occupational dispensing aims to provide a practical approach of promoting the concept of healthy sight now and healthy sight in future. The most crucial part to the implementation of the principles of occupational dispensing is an awareness of the relationship between vision care provider and vision wear. The real success relies upon the fact how well the provider explains and how well the wearer understands.

POINTS TO REMEMBER

- The primary aim of occupational dispensing is to enhance the visual performance for the specific occupation.
- While providing the solution the optician must explain the benefits and advantage of the prescribed solution—what he will be gaining if he uses and what he will be missing if he does not use.
- Swimming sunglasses are used for surface swimming only.
- Half eye frames are very effective for reading in supine position.
- Occupational lenses are specific purpose lenses that cannot be used for general purpose.

DIGITAL DISPENSING SYSTEMS AND LENS CUSTOMIZATION

Digitization is the process of converting information into a digital format. It allows information to be looked at from the wider perspective. Digital Dispensing is the use of an integrated, computer-based system comprised of simulation, 3-dimensional visualization, analytics and various collaboration tools to measure multiple dispensing measurements to incorporate measured data in lens manufacturing to enhance the lens performance. The objective of Chapter 15 is to highlight the application of modern digital dispensing measuring systems and explain how customization of lenses can improve visual performance of the lenses.

Digital dispensing system—the current trend of optical dispensing is a revolutionary technology that provides advanced fitting and measurement system with patient consultation in one simple process. It is totally a computer driven technology that allows following facilities:

- Measures various dispensing measurements.
- Demonstrates the use and application of various lens types.
- Allows the customer to select a suitable lens matching to his prescription.
- Facilitates frame selection.
- Allows the patient to make a complete informed decision.

The new technology replaces the old traditional optician rulers, pupillometer and Y-Stick that were used to take dispensing measurements. It includes fully integrated, computer-based system that comprises of simulation, 3-dimensional visualization and various other tools that provides inputs on various dispensing measurements in the form of numerical data. These data are transferred to sophisticated generators to process most precise high definition lenses.

The technology allows the optician to capture precisely:

- Interpupillary distance for each eye separately.
- Exact position of the segment heights and fitting cross position.
- Pantoscopic tilt of the spectacle frame on the wearer's face.

- Face form wrap of the spectacle frame on the wearer's face.
- Vertex distance.

In addition the technology also allows to capture various biometric data like head-eye movement ratio, habitual reading distance, habitual reading posture and dominant eye that can be combined with patient's prescription and a unique digitally customized lens can be produced that optimizes the performance of the lens on eyes and gives the wearer a total personalized viewing experience. Visioffice from Essilor, Zeiss's RV Terminal and Impression IST by Rodenstock are some of the popular digital system that provide all essential dispensing functions. Besides they also create photo images of the probable output that may be reviewed by the patient and dispenser both to make an informed decision. An interactive demonstration of lenses and lens enhancements is the additional feature that makes lens dispensing lot easier. The immediate benefits that can be seen are:

- More patient satisfaction.
- Facilitates premium lens sales.
- Facilitates customized lens dispensing.
- Makes you and your practice different from others.

Modern sophisticated lens designs offer unsurpassed optical performance. However, the actual benefits of those lenses are possible only by the accuracy of their fitting and dispensing. Digital dispensing system makes the life easier by consistently delivering the most precise measurements to ensure that the patient receives the best possible visual performance from these lenses. For the first time the lens designer gets those information in absolute terms and incorporate the same in lens manufacturing system so that they can really achieve their desired goal of providing high visual performance. The new digital dispensing system is capable of capturing several new measurements which were never taken before to allow lens manufacturer to provide real high definition lenses. Besides, the new digital system also allows the opticians to demonstrate and answer various questions that were never answered because of limitations of demonstration tools and complexities of optics, thus removing uncertainties, puzzling and frustrating experiences from the dispensing process. Now with these new digital dispensing systems the opticians can demonstrate:

1. Expected lens thickness.
2. Antireflection coating affectivity
3. Changing tint profile of photochromatic lenses
4. Look of the frame
5. Lens performance simulations.

The differing skills of multiple employees in busy stores also add confusions and difficulties. The new digital dispensing system allows easier and more automated dispensing measurements that improve accuracy and consistency to reduce fitting times and fitting errors. Fortunately, the new generation digital dispensing technology is a great help to opticians to allay their customers' concerns by making the dispensing process more precise, more personal, more enjoyable and ultimate. Along with the "wow" reaction these new systems typically elicit from the patients, they are often favorably impressed with the high-tech look and feel of the dispensing system itself. Obtaining these via digital pictures are easy and make both the dispensary and laboratory better partners in the visual performance delivered to the patient. It also transforms the way in which frames and lens options can be demonstrated to the patients, enabling "try before you buy" experience. Digital dispensing systems are important to dispense customized lenses that are tailored to individual visual and lifestyle needs because they are the most effective tools available to capture unique visual needs of a person.

ESSILOR'S VISIOFFICE

Essilor's Visioffice system is the most innovative digitalized dispensing tool (Fig. 15.1). It can be utilized at all stages of dispensing process—frame selection, product recommendation, education and measurements. The system allows to measure live 3-dimensional measurement of human eye in the office quickly and accurately. This dynamic 3-dimensional measurement determines the exact space or position of eye rotation center (ERC). The ERC is the new reference for pupillary distance and fitting height measurement and what was an approximate vertex distance is now replaced by the distance between the ERC and the lens called eye rotation center distance (ERCd). These 3-dimensional measurements PD, fitting height and the ERCd build the very unique code of each eye, known as eyecode data which forms the foundation of the lens individualization based on the physiology of each wearer. Every person, every eye has its own code—the eyecode. With Essilor's Visioffice it can be captured accurately quickly and easily.

When directing the eyes to view a given object, all fixation axes will pass through the ERC and intercept the lens in the precise area. Knowing the position of the ERC is the only way to calculate the unique optical function for each gaze direction and achieve

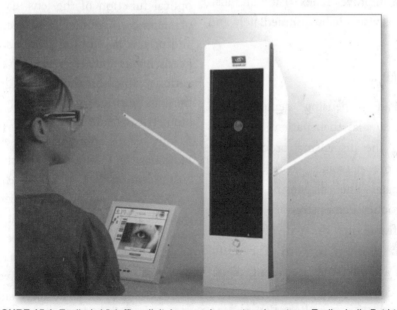

FIGURE 15.1: Essilor's Visioffice digital measuring system (courtesy: Essilor India Pvt Ltd)

the perfect lens to eye alignment. Rather than applying theoretical values, eyecode lenses are uniquely manufactured using mean 3-dimensional coordinates of ERC. When these very specific measurements are applied in the lens centering and lens manufacturing process, the patient gets the most precise vision instantly and effortlessly. With eyecode the patient receives the most uniquely designed lens that performs every time in all gaze direction.

Visioffice also captures pantoscopic tilt, face form wrap and several biometrical data that include head-eye movement ratio, habitual reading distance and sighting dominant eye of the wearer. Knowing these new measurements and visual behavioral information and incorporating them in the lens manufacturing process provide the unique lens design to an individual wearer that improves reflex vision and also adapts to his visual habits immediately and effortlessly.

NIKON'S IPAD

Nikon's iPad dispensing demonstration helps optician allay their patient's concerns by making the dispensing process more precise, more personal, more enjoyable and ultimate. The dispensing optician can do product demonstration, including how the frame fits the patient and the position in which it is worn. The useful features of Nikon's iPad are taking digital photos of consumers trying on their new eyewear and then emailing the photos,

or demonstrating premium lens options. Besides, demonstration of antireflection lenses, demonstration of changing tint of lenses indoors or outdoors and thickness comparison of various high-indices are also possible. The most amazing application of the system is lens simulation option that provides the option to the wearer to check how various new lifestyle and occupational lenses would cater his unique visual needs. Nikon iPad can also be used to educate the patient about basic ocular conditions. When attached with additional measuring attachment the system allows capturing various dispensing measurements also.

LENS CUSTOMIZATION

The dictionary meaning of customization is "to build or fit to an individual's specifications or needs or preferences". Customization of ophthalmic lens attempts to optimize the optical function of the lens, using variety of spherical, cylinder, aspherical surfaces and prisms based on an individual's visual needs, habits and preferences. In the process various anatomical factors that define the lens position in front of the eyes and biometric data are taken into considerations to improve the optics of the lenses on eyes. Flowchart 15.1 shows the objectives of lens customization.

All lenses can be customized for an individual patient whether it is single vision, bifocals or progressives addition lenses. Currently the lens manufacturers are keen on customizing progressive addition lenses. Some of the customized single vision lenses are also available. True customization

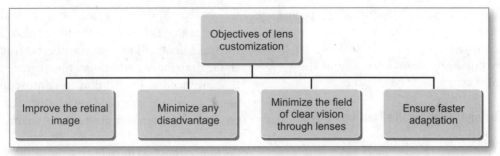

FLOWCHART 15.1: Objectives of lens customization

needs all those factors should be taken into consideration while lens designing that may affect the lens performance on wearer's eyes. On the wearer's eyes the performances of lenses are also influenced by:

1. Optical factors
2. Anatomical factors
3. Biometrical factors.

Optical factor requires an understanding of unique lens form based on refraction of the individual patient. The extension of the concept is various lens forms are adjudged against associated aberration profile that degrades the image quality to achieve the desired goal.

Anatomical factors require an understanding of the spectacle lens position that is defined by pantoscopic angle, panoramic angle and vertex distance of the eyewear on the patient's face. These are important fitting parameters that vary because of variation in structures of eyes, ears, nose and cheeks, and also with frame styles, shape and size.

Biometrical factors relate to individual's visual needs and developed visual habits like head and eye movements, head posture, habitual reading distance and dominant eye. A well-designed lens will always aim to establish the natural habit so as to minimize the strain on extra ocular muscles and ease binocular function during down gaze.

Currently lens customization is more common in progressive addition lenses. Lens manufacturers customize progressive addition lenses with respect to several factors that are shown in Flowchart 15.2.

Customization for the Prescription

The customization works only within the field of viewing zones, not allowing the zones to shrink because of oblique astigmatism

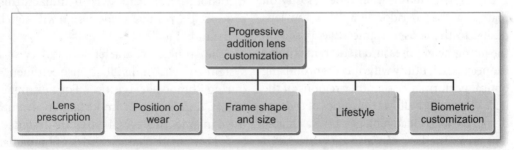

FLOWCHART 15.2: Progressive addition lens customization

that may be the result of inappropriate base curve selection. The process works to improve the optics of central viewing zones by providing more flexibility to choose the most appropriate base curve.

Customization for the Position of Wear

The actual position of spectacle frame determines the performance of lenses on eyes in real life. There are predominantly 3 important dynamics that explain the position of the spectacle frame on wearer's face. Pantoscopic tilt determines the lens position in vertical plane, face form wrap determines the lens position in horizontal plane and vertex distance determines effective lens power. They alter the visual performance of the lens by introducing oblique astigmatism resulting in an increase in sphere power and unwanted cylinder power. The selected frame is adjusted on the wearer's face and all measurements for aforesaid 3 dynamics are captured and incorporated while lens designing and compensated lens prescription is calculated, that improves the optical performance of the central viewing region of the lens on the wearer's face.

Customization for the Shape and Size of Frame

Frame style customization relies mostly on matching the corridor length of the lens design to the chosen frame style, based on the fitting height measurement to maximize the near vision utility without compromising optical performance on other regions of the lens. The process allows the optics of the lens design to take full advantage of the available lens area. The lens can also be customized to the shape of the frame. Lenses designed for wrap sports frames are typically compensated for shape of the frame also. "A" measurement, "B" measurements and frame shape drawing are additional measurements that are needed in addition to pantoscopic angle, face form wrap and vertex distance to customize the lens for given frame shape.

Customization for Lifestyle

Assessing the relative visual demands between distance and near viewing zones of the lens design is the key. Relevant information may be captured using a questionnaire of some form. Lens prescription may provide important clues for lifestyle customization. Lifestyle customizations are very effective to minimize immediate dissatisfaction.

Biometric Customization

Visual behavioral studies for eye and head movement reveals that a predominant eye mover will see differently as compare to a predominant head mover while fixating through a point other than the optical center of the lens. The eye mover uses more of the physical surface of the lens, whereas the head mover uses more of the central portion of the lens during dynamic vision. These variations in visual behavioral can be captured in numerical values using digital dispensing measuring systems and can be incorporated in the lens manufacturing process. The resultant lens design will match to the individual's visual habits.

The innate characteristics of visual system of an individual also influence during binocular vision. For example, ocular dominance is important in driving the dynamics of 2 eyes. Lenses are designed, based on innate characteristics of binocular vision system works very effectively to improve reflex visual performance of an individual. The pair of the lens works for the pair of eyes.

Besides, habitual reading distance and habitual reading posture are also important data to design lenses to suit the wearer's habit so that the lens is adapted to him quickly and effortlessly. The design philosophy aims to improve possibility of fast adaptation and minimize the disadvantage that a wearer may feel, such as swimming effect during adaptation period.

The transfer of new cutting—edge "free-form technology" to the patient is probably the biggest challenge for the dispensing optician. The design and manufacture of prescription ophthalmic lenses have really been a compromise between good optics, cosmetic considerations, tools and machinery limitations and inventory concerns. In fact, the lenses that had been manufactured with traditional surfacing methods were providing corrections for prescriptions but uncorrected for optical aberrations and other mechanical limitations. The new free-form technology has enabled the lens manufacturer to optimize the lens design to overcome optical aberrations and mechanical limitations of traditional surfacing. The new technology enhances precision in lens manufacturing and provides opportunity to incorporate personalization of lens designing. In order to achieve the desired results of the new free-form high definition lenses, there is a need of certain additional dispensing measurements that may include:

1. Pantoscopic angle of the spectacle frame.
2. Panoramic angle of the spectacle frame.
3. Vertex distance.
4. Boxing measurements of spectacle frames.
5. Visual behavior measurements.
6. Postural measurements.

Most often these measurements remain unattainable until the introduction of new digital dispensing measurements systems. Combining these data with the patient's prescription enables the optical laboratory to produce a lens that optimizes the performance of the lens and gives the wearer a totally personalized viewing experience.

POINTS TO REMEMBER

- The new digitalized dispensing system have transformed the way in which frames and lens options can be demonstrated to the patients, enabling "try before you buy" experience.
- The new digital dispensing system is capable of capturing several new measurements which were never taken before to allow lens manufacturer to provide real high definition lenses.
- Essilor's Visioffice system can be utilized at all stages of dispensing process—frame selection, product recommendation, education and measurements.
- Eyecode data can be captured accurately quickly and easily with Essilor's Visioffice.
- Lens customization aims to improve the retinal image quality.
- Customization of progressive addition lenses for prescription improves the optical performance of central viewing region of the progressive addition lenses.
- Customization of progressive addition lenses for position of wear minimizes the disadvantages that may occur because of the lens position on patient's eyes.

LENS ORDERING AND VERIFICATIONS

The purpose of Chapter 16 is to set a standard process and defined terminology that can be used to order lenses to lens laboratory and also to verify lenses with lens prescription. The onus is to use uniform terminology and checklist to ensure minimum error and improve quality control procedure.

Lens ordering and verification of lenses are backend job for optical dispensing. The process of lens ordering starts after all measurements are taken and all necessary documentations are completed that establishes a contractual relation between the patient and the optician. The process of lens ordering may be manual or totally computerized. However, there is a need for standardized protocols and procedures to maintain consistency and minimize errors.

LENS ORDERING

When the order for spectacle is confirmed the dispensing optician needs to procure the lenses from the lens manufacturer. It is important that all the lenses that are ordered, should be in writing either in soft copy or in hard copy. The optician may use his own format or may use the manufacturer's prescribed form. Each lens order should be given in separate sheet or form. Poor handwriting or illegible handwriting may result in error. When the order is given to have the ready spectacle in hand, relevant frame should also be sent together with the order. Only required information should be filled up in the order form. Unnecessary or superfluous information must be avoided. These are all very important to avoid errors in processing. All information that is needed may be grouped in 4 categories as shown in the Flowchart 16.1.

Lens Information

The lens material needs to be selected between mineral glass lens and organic plastic lens, and other information needed pertaining to lenses as stated in Flowchart 16.2 should be provided.

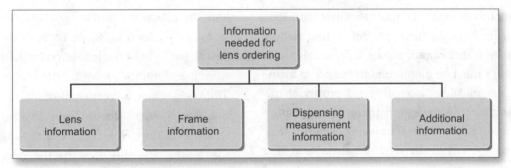

FLOWCHART 16.1: Important information needed for lens ordering

However, care must be taken to provide correct information as follows:

1. While writing the lens power, always write data for right eye first and then write data for left eye. Always use 3 digits for sphere and cylinder component. If the dioptric unit is less than 1.00 D, do not forget to use 0 before the decimal point. The lens power must be written with plus or minus sign. Mention the axis with prefatory '@' or 'X' and do not put degree sign after the numbers representing axis value as it may be read for an extra 0.

2. In case the lens prescription also shows prism, the required prism diopter has to be mentioned with its base direction.

3. If any type of lens coating is needed, it should be mentioned categorically as required by the laboratory. Do not forget to mention the tint, if needed. Tint may be solid or gradient, the darkness of which may be mentioned as percentage of light transmission. For example, indoor use tint are usually LT 80, whereas tint for sunglass may be LT 20 or less. Attaching a tint sample or mentioning the tint code of the manufacturer avoids all miscommunication related issues.

4. In case a specific lens brand is needed, a clear instructions must be given about the brand name and need for "Certificate of Authenticity". A brand savvy patient would never accept the lens without "Certificate of Authenticity".

Frame Information

In case the ordered lens is to be cut and fitted by the lens manufacturer, frame has to be

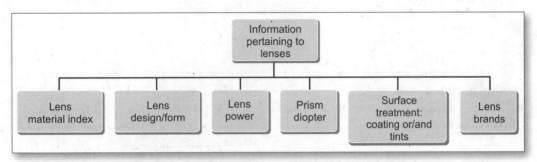

FLOWCHART 16.2: Important information pertaining to lenses

sent to the manufacturer together with lens order form. In such case detail information as to frame brand, model number, size and color must be mentioned in the order form. Care must be taken to send proper shape and size of the lens if there is any change needed for rimless frame. A sample lens may be cut in the required shape and size for the purpose.

Dispensing Measurement Information

Flowchart 16.3 shows the information pertaining to dispensing measurement that are very important to supply to the laboratory for dispensing lenses correctly.

1. Measure the effective diameter of lens needed in millimeter to cut the lens so that it encompasses the full longest diameter of the frame. In order to measure effective diameter mark the positions of the monocular interpupillary distance (IPD) on the lens insert that shows the position of optical center. Now measure the distance from the position of optical center of the lens to the apex of the lens bevel farthest from it and multiply it by 2. It allows maintaining the optical center correctly and ensure thinner lens edge profile. For progressive addition lens the effective diameter is measured from the position of fitting cross of the lens to the apex of the lens bevel farthest from it and multiply it by 2.

2. Thickness issue is very important not only for cosmetic reasons but also for wearing comfort. However, while making the lenses, we only look at the edge thickness, which is the result of resultant center thickness (CT). When lenses were hand-edged high minus glass lenses were made with a minimum CT of 0.6 mm. But with the introduction of modern auto edger where lenses are clamped by their center, the minimum CT for glass lens was increased to 1.00 mm to avoid lens shattering from stress. As a general rule, the CT varies from 2 mm down to 1 mm—the value decreasing as power increases. While ordering lenses for supra and rimless frames an extra thickness is considered specially in case of lower lens prescription. The width of the supra grooving is usually between 0.55–1.20 mm wide and the depth of the grooving varies from 0.20 mm to 1.0 mm deep. The shape is usually "U"

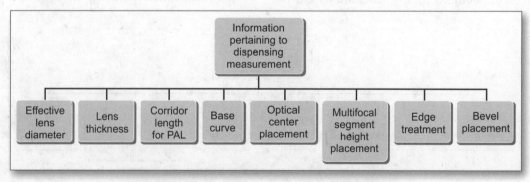

FLOWCHART 16.3: Dispensing measurement information

shaped groove. In case of plus lens, edge thickness is very important to ensure adequate width of supra grooving.

3. The choice of corridor length of progressive lens may vary between 10–21 mm depending upon specific lens design and "B" measurement of the frame. The associated factors that need to be understood before ordering for a particular corridor length are "minimum fitting height" and "recommended fitting height" for a given progressive lens design. Some laboratories recommend minimum fitting height criteria. It is therefore, mandatory to gather all specific information pertaining to each lens brand and then place the order for specific progressive lens design. Ideally, while selecting the suitable corridor length care should be taken to ensure that "B" measurement of the frame allows to obey the "recommended fitting height" criteria and also allows for sufficient amount of clearance above the fitting cross.

4. Base curve of an ophthalmic lens is the starting point from where the remaining curves are calculated. Base curve of an ophthalmic lens varies not only for different ranges of power but also for the same range of power among different lens manufacturers. Usually the choice of suitable base curve is done by lens manufacturer. But there are certain cases when a patient is used to a particular base curve, and changing the base curve may not be a wise decision. In such cases while placing order for the lenses, specific required base curve must be mentioned. Base curve must be adjusted for change in refractive index of the material.

5. Measured IPD is important information that must be given. In case of single vision lenses for distance vision, mention the monocular values of IPD for each eye separately and in case of single vision lenses for near vision mention binocular IPD for near vision. The values of binocular IPD for near vision may be divided equally and used as reference point to place the optical center of the lens. For a segmented bifocal lens do not forget to mention IPD for both, distance vision and for near vision separately. Monocular distance PD is important for progressive addition lenses. Vertical placement of optical center should be mentioned either with reference to datum line or with reference to lower rim of the frame. Usual practice is to provide the vertical position of the optical center with reference to the datum line. When specifying the vertical position of optical center, it is acceptable to indicate how much above or below the datum line. In general optical center should be placed 3–4 mm below the pupil with the head erect for a frame with a pantoscopic tilt of 6–8° for single vision distance lenses. If the spectacle is intended for reading only, optical center can be placed little lower.

6. Horizontal and vertical position of the near segment of a multifocal lens is very important for successful dispensing of multifocal lenses. Binocular IPD for near is critical for horizontal placement of near segment of a segmented bifocal lens. Monocular IPD for distance is important for progressive addition lenses. Vertical

positioning of near segment is measured either with reference to datum line or with reference to lower rim of the frame. Segment height as measured should be mentioned in millimeter either from lower rim of the frame or above and below datum line. In case there is a difference between vertical heights for right eye and left eye, do not forget to stress upon this fact.

7. Bevel placement is very critical when the lenses are thicker because of higher lens prescription. Flat bevel may obstruct while making nose pads adjustments in case of metal frames. Bevel placement may be specified as all forward, or 1/3rd forward or 2/3rd forward and should be equally protruded from outside in both eyes. Be careful as all forward placement of bevel shifts the entire lens thickness behind the frame eyewire. It is, therefore, important information to disguise the lens thickness.

8. Edge treatments are effective way to disguise lens thickness and make the spectacle lens appear cosmetically good. Decorative faceting to the edge of the lens, rubbing graphite pencil lead all over edge and polishing the lens edge before mounting the lenses into the frame are very effective to minimize reflections of edges at the lens surface.

Additional Information

Any additional information that forms the important part of either dispensing or delivery should also be given while placing the order for lenses. Date of delivery, modifications needed in bridge width specially for zyl frames, specialized packaging, etc. may be some of the important information.

LENS VERIFICATIONS

When the ready spectacles are received from the prescription laboratory, it is essential to verify them for following:

- **Color uniformity**: Lenses should be checked for color uniformity for right and left lenses. A broad view inspection against a white light box can help detect even subtle difference in color.
- **Bubbles**: The lens material must meet very high standards of purity. They must be free of bubbles, striae, stone and other defects. These defects are more common with mineral glass material and could interfere with light transmission or refraction. These defects can be easily detected by inspecting the lenses below bulb light.
- **Accuracy of the lens power**: Geneva Lens Measure, Lensometer or Neutralization technique may be applied to verify the lenses for the accuracy of lens power.
- **Optical center**: Lensometer may be used to verify the position of optical center.
- **Multifocal segment positioning**: The position of the near segment may be easily inspected below bulb light.
- **Lens thickness**: A broad view inspection for edge thickness and measuring the CT using caliper can provide fairly good information about the thickness profile of the lenses.
- **Lens insertion**: Make sure that the lenses are inserted well within the frame rim and the lens bevel is well-placed within the frame inside groove.
- **Frame fitting and alignment**: Make sure that the spectacle frame is adjusted properly and all aspects of standard alignment of frame is respected.

Progressive addition lenses contains a number of permanent microengravings and temporary ink markings. Use these ink markings to verify correct dispensing of progressive addition lens. Ensure that the distance power viewing circle and near power viewing circle are within the frame shape and the fitting cross is correctly placed.

POINTS TO REMEMBER

- All lenses must be ordered in writing either in soft copy or in hard copy.
- Always mention the cylinder axis with prefix '@' or 'X' and do not put degree sign after the numbers representing axis value as it may be read for an extra 0.
- Base curve of an ophthalmic lens is the starting point from where the remaining curves are calculated.
- Bevel placement is very important to disguise the lens thickness within the frame eyewire.
- Edge treatments are effective way to disguise lens thickness and make the spectacle lens appear cosmetically appealing.
- Multifocal segment height is mentioned either with reference to lower eyewire or datum line.

LENS INSERTION

Different frame styles and different frame materials require different techniques for inserting lenses into the frames to ensure a neat and perfect end result. The purpose of Chapter 17 is to explain the step-by-step procedure involved in lens insertion.

Inserting lenses into frames is an art and it needs proper tools and equipments. The optician needs to have a complete working table and a trained fitter who can consistently perform the job. The working table should be fully equipped with all tools and equipments needed for lens insertion and other necessary materials used during fitting procedures. Spectacles frame warmers, screwdrivers, nut drivers, a set of specially designed pliers, vice, polishers, files, flat top platform, ultrasonic cleaners, stress tester and pad popper are some of the basic tools and equipments needed. In addition there are some consumables that should also be always available readily. Bonding agents, loose screw set, spare nose pads, nylon threads, nail polish and edge markers are common amongst them.

LENS INSERTION INTO ZYL FRAMES

The entire process for lens insertion into zyl frame can be grouped under 3 broad heads:
1. Preparations
2. Insertion
3. Post fit inspection.

Preparations

1. Arrange heating unit, a bowl filled with water, a set of screwdrivers, a wiping cloth and tissue papers on a working table with adequate light on top.
2. Air blower, salt pan, hot water tub, warm heater and infrared heater may be used as heating unit as different materials respond differently to system of heating. Polycarbonate materials is the most difficult to soften for adjustment in a hotair frame heater. Nylon material frames cannot be heated uniformly enough by hot air or salt pan to allow stretching necessary for lens insertion. They tend to heat only outer layers of nylon while leaving the deeper portions

cool to stretch. Hot water penetrates the nylon better and allows stretching better to accept lenses. To heat nylon frame, heat the desired portion, bend as desired and then hold the frame in the new conformation while it is cooled. If you release before it is cooled, it tends to come back to its initial shape. Optyl material does not soften until the heat reaches 80°C, it can safely be heated at a level of 200°C without bubbling. Apply the heat at the desired point, gently insert the lens and then hold the same outside the water and allow it to cool down while holding. Do not plunge into the water to contract. It stops the shrinking process. Blower heater or salt pan may be effectively used for celluloid nitrate and celluloid acetate frames.

3. Detach the temples from the frame front before inserting the lens into the plastic frame front. It is quite likely that the weight of the temple may misalign or loosen the hinge when endpieces of the frame are heated and if the hinges are implanted into the front of the frame without front shield, it is possible that heat might weaken the hinge bonding.

4. Put a large cloth on your lap to prevent lens damaging if lens falls off your hand while inserting into the frame.

5. Compare the curvature of the lens meniscus as compared to the curve of the eyewire.

Insertion

1. Now you are ready for inserting the lens into the frame front. (Fig. 17.1)

2. Before you apply heat to the frame front, hold the lens in your hand at an angle and position that allows you to insert the lens immediately on heating. This is important to ensure minimum time lag after the frame is heated because zyl frames cool very rapidly and lose their pliability instantly.

3. If the lens curvature is more than the eyewire curve, it is advisable to apply little heat and reshape the upper and lower sections of the eyewire so that it conforms to the meniscus of the lens edge.

4. Now the frame is ready for lens insertion. Apply uniform heat to the eyewire from all around and make sure that the thicker portions, i.e. nasal and temporal eyewires are heated little more. Care should be taken to heat both the front and back of the eyewire alternately to avoid overheating while using air blower. The salt bath contains 2 components— salt and talcum powder. Salt conveys heat while talcum powder prevents salt from lumping and sticking to the frame. When the salt pan is used, make sure that you stir the salt to equalize the temperature and then push some of the salt into a mound in one portion of the pan. Place the section of the frame to be heated just beneath the salt mound as parallel to the surface of the salt as possible. Remember to place only the section that is to be heated, leaving the rest out of the salt. Move the frame continually and very slowly while under the salt to avoid salt granule sticking to dry frame. If salt sticks to a dry frame, additional talcum powder should be added to the salt. If you are using warm heater, keep moving the frame front in such a manner that the heat is applied to back, front and

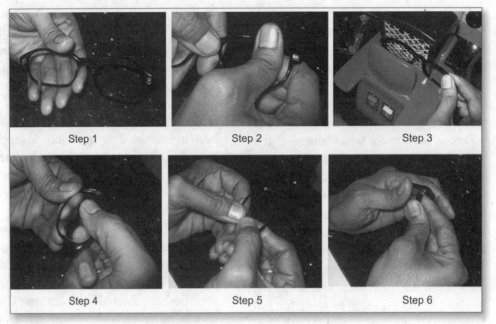

FIGURE 17.1: Sequential steps for lens insertion in plastic frame

entire eyewire uniformly. Keep checking the pliability of the eyewire by curving the eyewire to prevent overheating.

5. Now push the lens into the front eyewire. Insert the temporal edge of the lens into the outer edge of the frame from the back. Thumbs on the back surface of the lens and fingers on the nasal edge of the frame eyewire, snap the lens into the frame from the nasal side by pressure of both thumbs and fingers. If the frame has pads, take care not to bend or break it. Alternately, insert the upper temporal edge of the lens into the frame groove from the front, then push the lens holding it from the nasal edge into the eyewire so that the entire edge of the lens is in the frame.

6. Finally pull the lower portion of the eyewire around the lower lens edges. After inserting the lenses into the frame, plunge the frame and lenses into ice water to "set" them except when the frame material is optyl, as this can have exactly the opposite effect on lens tightness.

The following care must be taken while inserting the lens into the frame:

1. Make sure that there are no marks made by the lens against the softened plastic or by undue stretching of the plastic.

2. If the frame cools down before the lens is inserted fully, it is advisable to remove the lens totally before reheating the frame.

3. While pulling the eyewire, care must be taken that your pulling force is straight and make sure that the eyewires are not rolled out. The rolling of the eyewire will turn the groove at an angle, and will spoil the front appearance of the frame. A rolled eyewire does not secure the lens

tightly that results in constant complain of lens falling out of the frame front.

4. If the lower eyewire is rolled forward, i.e. front side is slanted down and in spite of all attempts to straighten it, it still remains a problem, reinsert the lens from back side of the frame.

Post Fit Inspection

1. Make sure that the lens is entirely placed in the groove of the eyewire.
2. The grooves of the eyewire are not rolled out. Be sure that the lens fits squarely from all around.
3. Make sure that the frame is not twisted from the bridge.
4. In case of flat top bifocal lens fitting, make sure both right and left top segment line are on same height and the segment edges are at similar distance from the nasal eyewire.

LENS INSERTION INTO SUPRA FRAMES

The entire process for lens insertion into supra frame can be grouped under 3 broad heads:

1. Preparations
2. Insertion
3. Post fit inspection.

Preparations

1. Supra frames, also known as rimlon frames or Nylor mounted frames use cord mounting for lens fitting. Arrange nylon monofilament cord, ribbon, a wiping cloth and tissue papers on a working table with adequate light on top.
2. Put a large cloth on your lap to prevent lens damaging if lens falls off your hand while inserting into the frame.

Insertion

1. Nylon monofilament cord is used to secure lenses to semi-rimless chassis. In order to fit the lens, the cord is attached to the mounting arm.
2. A groove is cut into the lens edge. This groove is the channel into which the monofilament cord is fitted. (Fig. 17.2)
3. The lens is inserted into the loop created by the monofilament cord using a ribbon to pull the line around the lens circumference. They secure the lenses completely around like a rim but without dealing with screws, hex nuts, filing, messy glues or special riveting tools and mounting pins.
4. The cord is susceptible to temperature change and can shrink over time and snap, but it can be easily changed.

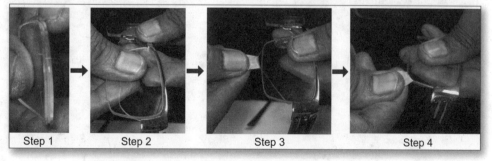

Step 1   Step 2   Step 3   Step 4

FIGURE 17.2: Sequential steps for lens insertion in supra frame

Post Fit Inspection

Make sure that the nylon monofilament run through the lens groove and is tightly attached to frame eyewire.

LENS INSERTION INTO RIMLESS FRAMES

Rimless frames are designed with no eyewire surrounding the lenses. Lenses are suspended and secured using several mounting methods including screws and hex nuts, fixing pins, bushing and cementing. The entire process for lens insertion into rimless frame differs with different types of mounting methods. Broadly, preparatory and post fit inspection stages remain the same, procedure of lens insertion differs.

Preparations

1. Arrange all accessories like screws, hex nuts, fixing pins, bushing, plastic washer and cementing glues together with a wiping cloth, and tissue papers on a working table with adequate light on top. In addition you also need some tools like a set of screwdrivers, a set of nut drivers, a set of pliers specially designed for rimless fitting, compression pliers, razor blade, cutting pliers, push pin and file.

2. Put a large cloth on your lap to prevent lens damaging if lens falls off your hand while inserting into the frame.

Insertion

The mounting of lenses using screws and nuts begins with drilling holes through the lenses and then follows the following process (Fig. 17.3):

1. First lens is placed on the mounting.
2. Screws are inserted through each hole.
3. Nuts are used to secure the lens in place.
4. This process is repeated for the second lens.
5. Excess screw length is cut away with cutter pliers and filed smooth.
6. A plastic washer may be used under the screw's head to cushion the pressure on the lens front and a plastic bushing may be used around the screw for the same purpose laterally.

The new compression technology, rimless mounting uses prongs on the bridge and endpieces which have barbs on them and special bushings that fit over them securely. Compression mounting technology is simple and is less stressful than screws and nuts. The plastic bushing not only secures the lenses but cushions

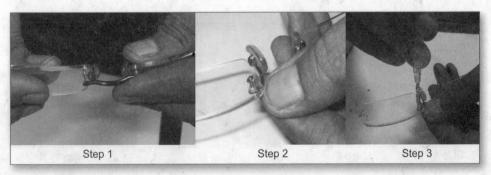

FIGURE 17.3: Sequential steps for lens insertion in screw mounting rimless frame

lateral lens movement which is important in reducing lens cracking around the drilled holes. The mounting of lenses begins with drilling holes through the lenses based on the manufacturers supplied layout chart and then follows the following process (Fig. 17.4):

1. Notch the lens if needed. Notch allows preventing post fit lens rotation, helping to keep the lens on axis.
2. Insert the bushings into the drilled holes through the backside of the lens.
3. Using a razor or cutting pliers, cut off the excess bushing so that it is flush with the outside surface of the lens.
4. Use a pushpin to reshape and reopen the tip of the bushing by gently inserting the tip into the opening.
5. Begin with one lens at a time at the bridge. From the front, insert the nasal prong into the nasal drill hole.
6. Place the front jaw of the compression pliers over the bridge and the opposite jaw onto the head of the bushing on the

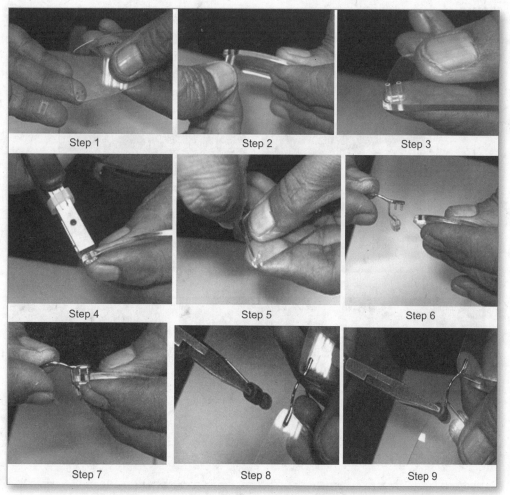

FIGURE 17.4: Sequential steps for lens insertion in compression technology rimless frame

backside of the lens. Slowly squeeze the plier's jaws to seat the bridge.

7. Fit the other end of the bridge to the other lens in the same way.

8. Repeat the above step for each endpiece.

Post Fit Inspection

1. Make sure that the lenses are securely mounted.

2. Extra length of screws is cut and a plastic cap is put on the screw end.

LENS INSERTION INTO FULL RIM METAL FRAMES

The entire process for lens insertion into full rim metal frame can be grouped under 3 broad heads:

1. Preparations
2. Insertion
3. Post fit inspection.

Preparations

1. Arrange all accessories like spare screws, cementing glues together with a wiping cloth and tissue papers on a working table with adequate light on top. In addition you also need some tools like a set of screwdrivers and a set of pliers.

2. Put a large cloth on your lap to prevent lens damaging if lens falls off your hand while inserting into the frame.

Insertion

1. Before inserting the lenses into metal frame make sure that meniscus curve of

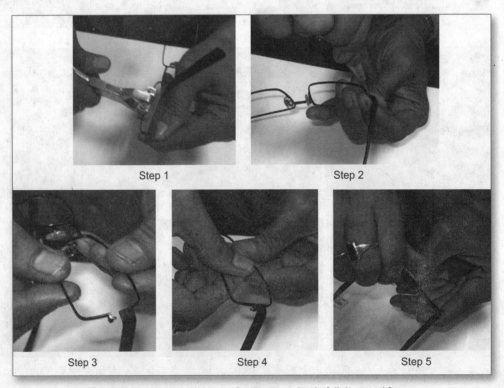

Step 1   Step 2   Step 3   Step 4   Step 5

FIGURE 17.5: Sequential steps for lens insertion in full rim metal frame

the top and bottom of the lens matches to the upper and lower eyewire of the frame front (Fig. 17.5).

2. If there is any mismatch the lens will not fit squarely in the eyewire groove. It means using eyewire forming pliers to reshape the eyewire rim is important.

3. Now remove the eyewire screws completely, put the lens within the eyewire and replace the eyewire.

4. Do not simply loosen the screws and put the lenses. It may cause lens chipping.

Post Fit Inspection

Make sure that the lenses are securely mounted.

POINTS TO REMEMBER

- Hot water is the best way to heat the nylon frames for lens insertion.
- If salt from the salt pan sticks to the frame, add talcum powder to the salt to alleviate the problem.
- Optyl frame may be heated until they bend under their own weight.
- Polycarbonate materials is the most difficult to soften for adjustment in a hotair frame heater.
- Nylon monofilament cord is used to secure lenses to semi-rimless chassis.
- Lenses are suspended and secured using several mounting methods including screws and hex nuts, fixing pins, bushing and cementing.

FITTING SPECTACLE FRAME

Optical dispensing is also an art to fit the spectacle frame snugly on the patient's face so that it makes contact with the face comfortably and serves its purpose to his satisfaction. Proper adjustments of frame are crucial for the purpose. A fine sense of observation and touch is an attribute of a good dispensing optician. You need to remember that every patient has different anomalies and you are fitting a spectacle frame to ensure comfort for the patient, not a flat surface for square or for pretty look only. Chapter 18 acquaints the readers with the art of observing the frame fitting on the patient's face and then making necessary adjustments to ensure that the frame is fitted to the patient comfortably.

Optical dispensing is an art. The art entails that all the important aspects of spectacle frame fitting on the wearer's face should be checked and required alteration is being done before asking the patient to undergo a short adaptation period. Spectacle frame rests on the nose and is held in place by temples extending through the sides of the face towards or over the ears of the wearer such that the wearer can wear it comfortably for a longer period of time and can enjoy perfect vision. A well-fitted spectacle frame will always fit snugly to be most comfortable and will always look good and serve its true function, whereas an ill-fitted spectacle frame would be the reason for dissatisfaction.

A well-fitted spectacle frame implies that the different aspects of frame fitting as shown in Flowchart 18.1 has been taken care of for an individual concerned.

PANTOSCOPIC ANGLE

Pantoscopic angle is the angle between the temples of the frame near joints and the superior rim of the front of the frame as shown in Figure 18.1. The top of the frame front lies away from the eyebrows and the bottom of the frame front moves towards the cheeks, creating a parallel relation with facial plane. Pantoscopic angle refers to the alignment of the frame in its up and down position. All the spectacle frames are designed to have a certain degree of pantoscopic angle which varies between the

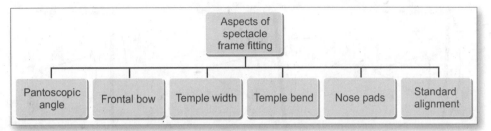

FLOWCHART 18.1: Different aspects of frame fitting

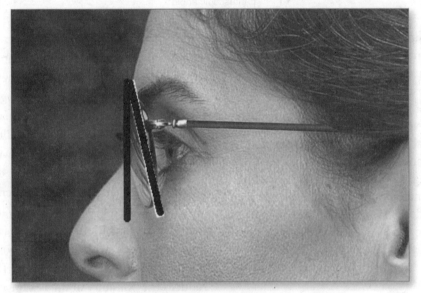

FIGURE 18.1: Pantoscopic angle

ranges of 4°–6° so that the spectacle frame rests parallel to the slope of the facial front. The angle between the temples and the frame front should never be vertical or 90°. Both the temples should be equally angled to the front of the frame. It divides the frame front on the wearer's face into 2 segments—the upper being used for distance vision and the lower being used for near vision. Thus it brings the near zone closer to the eyes and increases the field of view through the near zone of the lens.

Figures 18.2A to C show the different degree of pantoscopic angle. Retroscopic angle is the opposite to pantoscopic angle in which case the bottom of the eyewire of frame front sit out further from the face than the top of the eyewire, the temple is actually angled up and is away from the front. Retroscopic angle may be required on the people with full cheeks, but is never a desirable condition.

Effect of Pantoscopic Angle

Pantoscopic angle is an important fitting measurement that determines vertical position of the spectacle frame on the wearer's face. The effects of the tilt are noted as:

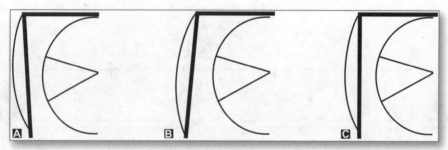

FIGURES 18.2 A to C: A. Positive pantoscopic angle, B. Negative pantoscopic angle/ retroscopic angle, C. No pantoscopic angle

1. It brings the near zone closer to the eyes and increases the field of view through the near zone of the lens. Inadequate pantoscopic tilt can reduce the effective size of the near zone.
2. For every 2° of pantoscopic angle, the optical center for distance drops down by 1 mm.
3. Tilting a spherical lens causes oblique astigmatism adding both spherical and cylinder of same sign of the original lens, with cylinder axis in the axis of the tilt (Fig. 18.3).

Significance

The curvature and tilt of the spectacle lenses are designed to minimize the astigmatism of oblique incidence. Pantoscopic tilt is the forward tilt of the spectacle plane relative to the vertical. If the spectacle lenses were perpendicular to the horizon, there would be significant astigmatism of oblique incidence in the reading position. If they were optimized for reading position, astigmatism of oblique incidence would be maximum for distance vision. Pantoscopic tilt of 4°–6° forward is a compromise between the optimal position of the lenses for distance and near work. In daily life we spend most of our time looking slightly downward from the primary position, and spectacles are therefore, made with the lower portion of the lens tilted towards the cheek. This also reduces the obliquity of the reading portion of multifocal lenses. However, it may be a cause of intolerance in high-power spectacle lenses if new frames are dispensed which have different angle of pantoscopic tilt from the wearer's previous spectacle frame.

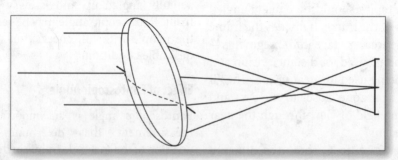

FIGURE 18.3: Tilting a lens causes the effect of oblique astigmatism

Advantage

1. This minimizes the effect of oblique astigmatism, an aberration that would be induced with down gaze if the lens were fitted perpendicular to the distance visual axis.
2. This also minimizes the vertex distance changes. Since the top of the lens is intentionally tilted forward, this helps to achieve a place that allows a more constant distance between the back surface of the lens and the front surface of the cornea.

Measuring Pantoscopic Tilt

Pantoscopic tilt is measured on the wearer's face from a vertical plane parallel to the face and perpendicular to the line of sight in the primary gaze. Specially designed tools like Zeiss Pendulum and Rodenstock Clip-On scale containing a ball bearing are available for the purpose. Put the spectacle frame on the wearer's face and ask him to look straight ahead and then use the Zeiss Pendulum device as shown in Figure 18.4. This device

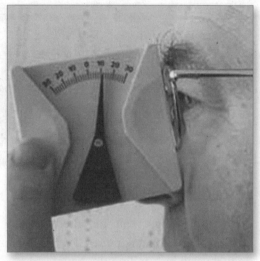

FIGURE 18.4: Zeiss Pendulum

offers great clarity of reading and ease of use, thus resulting in very effective and accurate measurement.

Rodenstock Clip-On scale containing a ball bearing is also very effective tool to measure pantoscopic angle. Nikon Measuring Scale (Fig. 18.5) is also very simple measuring device for the purpose.

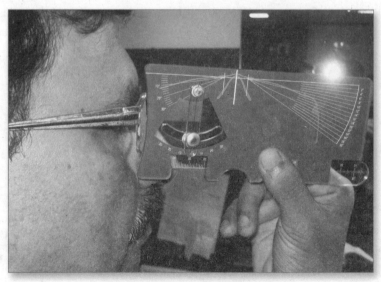

FIGURE 18.5: Nikon Measuring Scale

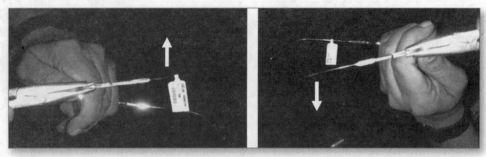

FIGURE 18.6: Angling metal frames

Altering Pantoscopic Tilt

Pantoscopic angle can be altered using angling plier for metal frames. The angle can be increased by bending the temples down from the frame front at the endpiece to increase the tilt, and by bending the temples up to decrease the pantoscopic angle as shown in Figure 18.6.

However, in case of plastic frame, apply heat around the endpiece from the frame front to soften the portion and then push down the portion taking temple together to increase the angle, and push up the portion taking temple together to decrease the angle.

FRONTAL BOW

Frontal bow, also known as face form wrap or dihedral angle or apical curve or angle of wrap is the measurement of the amount of bow on the front of the frame that is provided to ensure that the front of the frame follows the line of the wearer's face as seen from the top (Fig. 18.7). It can be provided from the 2 points on the frame front— eyewire rim and the bridge. The bridge of the frame sits slightly more forward than the endpieces. Frontal bow determines the angle at which the horizontal plane of the lens lies in relation to the horizontal plane of the face.

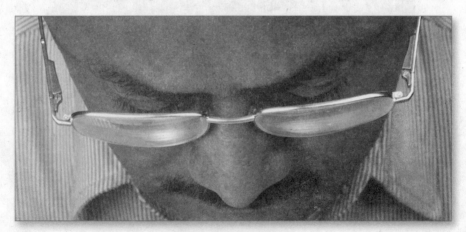

FIGURE 18.7: Frontal bow

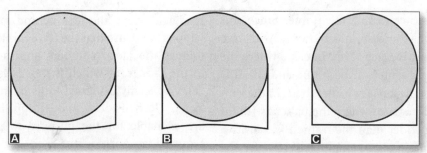

FIGURES 18.8 A to C: A. Positive face form, B. Negative face form, C. No face form

When a spectacle frame leaves the factory, it always carry a certain degree of face form wrap which may vary from 5° to 7° from the frame front plane. Like pantoscopic angle there may be three possibilities for face form wrap on the wearer's face as shown in Figures 18.8A to C.

Positive face form wrap (Fig. 18.8A) is the most desired in which case the frame front sits slightly more forward from the bridge than the endpieces of the frame. This is essential for both cosmetic and optical reasons.

Effect of Face Form Wrap

Positive face form wrap has great impact on the optical performance of the spectacle lenses, some of the most common effects are:

1. It brings the geometrical center of the frame nearer to the wearer's IPD, if the IPD of the wearer is smaller than the distance between the 2 geometric centers of the frame.
2. Ensures cosmetically acceptable look of frame on the wearer's face.
3. It also works as locking the spectacle frame on the wearer's face from temporal sides.
4. The optical effect of the face form wrap can be understood from the concept of wrap around sports lenses. Compared to standard curve lens a wrap sports lens is a steeper curve lens that tilts the lens in the vertical plane. The new configurations affect the wearer's vision, unless the optics of the lens is optimized for the effect of wrap. The primary optical effect is offset in the prism and power of the lens perceived by the wearer which may be objectionable specially in higher power. Even a plano wrap lens introduces prism. Fortunately the conventional spectacle lenses are not as wrapped as sports lenses. But similar effect may be noticed by the wearer in case of high power when excessive face form wrap is given to spectacle frame front.

Significance

The curvature and tilt of the spectacle frames are designed to minimize the effect of astigmatism of oblique incidence. In practice face form wrap of the frame is altered while mounting the lenses into them so that the lens stay fitted and do not come out, which is usually done from the eyewire rim and compensatory adjustments is done either from the bridge or from the endpieces. Positive face form wrap should be used when the patient's IPD is narrower than the geometric center of the frame. Since this is usually the case, most frames will have some positive face form. In cases where the geometric center of the frame and the IPD are the same, no face form is best. In the very unusual instance where the patient's IPD is actually wider than the frame PD, negative face form should be employed. However, the need to apply negative face form can usually be avoided with a more appropriate frame selection.

Advantages

1. Minimizes the vertex distance changes.
2. Ensures a cosmetically appealing and stable fit of spectacle frame on the wearer face.

Measuring Face Form Wrap

Measuring the face form wrap for a traditional spectacle frame is little different than measuring the same for a sports frame. While measuring the face form wrap for sports frame, the frame must be on the wearer's head because the spreading of sides as the frame passes over the temples tends to alter the effective wrap on face because of the width of the head. For a dress wear spectacle frame the idea behind providing wrap is to ensure that the frame front gently follows the facial contours and is parallel to the face front which is mostly less than 180°. Specially designed tools from Nikon, Zeiss, Rodenstock and Rupp+Hubrach are available for the purpose to measure required face form wrap.

Altering Face Form Wrap

While adjusting rimless frame for frontal bow use 2 pliers as shown in Figure 18.9 to provide face form wrap from bridge. Brace the position where the screw or bushing is inserted through the hole in the lens. Use the double nylon jaw gripping pliers to angle the bridge so that the curve is moved "inward" or as needed. Use 2 pliers to align lenses.

For plastic frame apply little heat at the bridge and then give desired curve as shown in Figure 18.10. Metal frames can also be bent from the bridge portion to apply frontal bow.

TEMPLE WIDTH

Temple width is the measure of the distance between the inner portions of one temple to

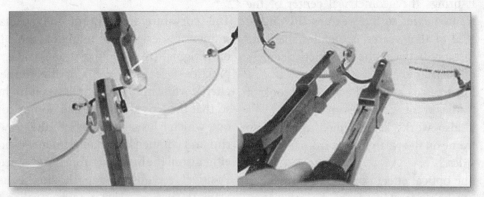

FIGURE 18.9: Adjusting rimless frame for frontal bow

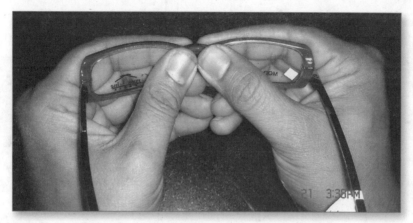

FIGURE 18.10: Applying frontal bow in plastic frames

inner portion of other temple of the frame as shown in Figure 18.11. It is measured at a level approximately 25–30 mm behind the spectacle frame front plane.

Measuring temple width per se is not very important for the dispensing optician. It has to be measured together with the measurement of the facial width of the wearer. Facial width implies the distance between the 2 temporal bones of the face at a level approximately 25–30 mm behind the nose crest plane around the ears as shown in Figure 18.12.

The 2 most important fittings associated with front and sides are the horizontal and the vertical angle of sides, that is being made with the front plane at joints. Horizontal angle relates to the angle of the let-back, i.e. angle between the inner surfaces of the fully opened temples that

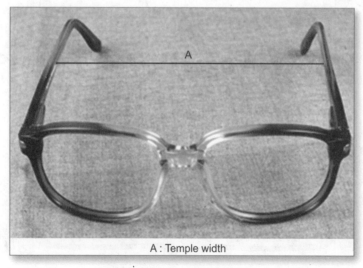

A : Temple width

FIGURE 18.11: Temple width of frame

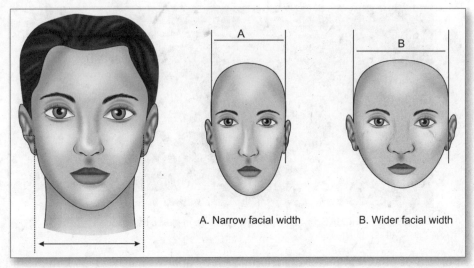

FIGURE 18.12: Facial width

are being formed with the plane of the front as shown in Figure 18.13. The angle of let-back determines the temple width of the spectacle frame. The larger angle of the let-back implies that the 2 temples are wide apart with increased temple width and the smaller let-back angle means the distance between the 2 temples at a level approximately 25–30 mm behind the spectacle frame front plane is narrow.

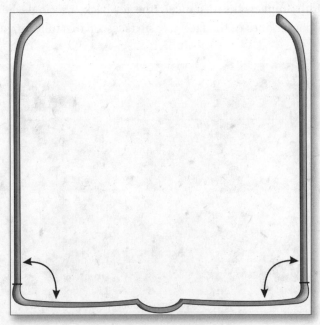

FIGURE 18.13: The angle of let-back

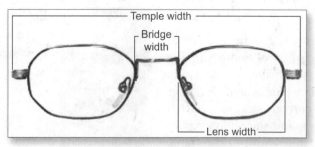

FIGURE 18.14: Temple width

When we measure the temple width without reference to facial width, it is taken to be sum of the measurement of bridge width plus width of the 2 lens size plus the width of endpieces of each side that hang out from the lens rim as shown in Figure 18.14. If the selected frame size matches to this distance, temple width ensures perfect fit on the wearer's face.

Effect of Temple Width

There are number of variations that can be seen as far as the shape of human skull is concerned. However, there is one unique aspect that is being observed commonly in most people, i.e. the anterior part of the head is wedge-shaped. The plane of the face normally represents the narrowest that gradually becomes the widest around the ear point and is followed by another wedge-shaped part of the skull that points away from the face as shown in Figure 18.15.

If the temple width of the frame is narrower than the facial width or in other words the angles of the let-back are too small, the wedge will become operational and the spectacle frame will have tendency to propel forward. Therefore, the measured temple width of the frame has to conform

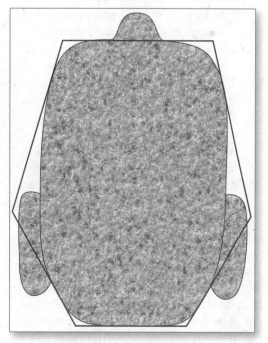

FIGURE 18.15: Wedge-shaped head

with facial width of the wearer so that the temples when running through the sides of the face makes parallel relation with the temporal bones and makes contact only on top of the ears. Both the temples of the frame should be equally angled out or angled in. If the right temple of the frame is angled out more than the left temple, it will cause the right side of the frame front to move in and vice versa.

Significance

The size of the frame selected should be in scale with the size of facial width. Smaller frame size will have smaller facial width, while larger facial width will have larger frame size. The correct size so selected should be fitted to follow the philosophy of fitting triangle. Temple width of the frame must be adjusted to the facial width in such a manner that it establishes a parallel relation with the sides of the face and makes contact with the temporal face around the ears only. A narrow temple width will result in:

1. The spectacle frame will propel forward, thereby it will increase vertex distance and alter the effect of lens prescription.
2. It does not allow the frame front to rest correctly on the nose crest.
3. It may create unsightly marks on the temporal skull.
4. It makes the spectacle frame uncomfortable to the wearer.

On the other hand, a very wide temple width as compare to the facial width will result in the spectacle fit that is loose on the wearer's face, and is characterized by the poor stability of the spectacle frame on the nose crest. Most complains like loose fit, tight fit, comfortable fit, uncomfortable fit, slipping or hurting, unsightly marks on nose and at the sides of temple bones and also some vision related complains can be managed by maneuvering temple width of the spectacle frame. It is, therefore, not wrong to say that the temple width of the frame is the most critical aspect of overall spectacle frame fitting.

Advantage

1. This is important to minimize the vertex distance changes as it ensures a stable fit of spectacle frame on the wearer's face.

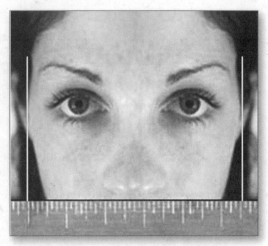

FIGURE 18.16: Measuring facial width

2. The temples of the frame do not create marks on the temple portion of the face.

Measuring Temple Width

The required temple width for a wearer is determined by measuring the facial width of the wearer. The simple millimeter rule may be used to measure the facial width of the wearer as shown in Figure 18.16.

Altering Temple Width

Modification in the temple width can be done from the endpieces. In order to modify the temple width of a rimless frame brace the mountings with double-side covered pliers and push the endpiece, inward or outward with flat or round pliers since the round post will not kink the metal as shown in Figure 18.17.

Temple width of metal frames can also be modified in the similar fashion. Brace the joint where endpiece is soldered with the eyewire using double-sided rubber pliers

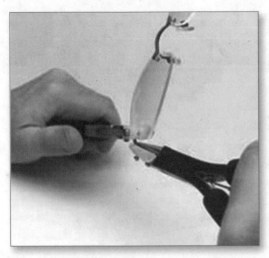

FIGURE 18.17: Altering temple width

and apply adequate pull or push to pull out or push in the temples from the joints. However, in case of plastic frames, there are 2 ways of altering the temple width:

1. Use a file to remove a small amount of the material from the temple top near the hinge (Fig. 18.18). But you cannot reduce the temple width using this method.

2. Another method is to apply heat around the endpiece of the frame front holding the frame in an angular position as shown in Figure 18.19. Then bend the lugs in, to decrease the temple width and bend the lugs out, to increase the temple width. Be careful not to do from the hinge portion which may damage the hinge.

Stretching out the temples to enclose the full facial width does not complete the adjustments; both the temples need to be curved to follow the shape of the temporal head as shown in the Figure 18.20.

Since the facial width is measured around the earpoint which is the widest portion of the skull and just beyond the earpoint there is a depression in the mastoid bone that varies in shape and size, the fitting adjustment of temple width requires that the ends of the temples must be bent inwards slightly to create parallel relation with the temporal head and keep the spectacle frame stable on the wearer head. The spectacle frame has to be fitted with features opposite to the shape of the face and facial bones to ensure stability. The straight forward meaning is

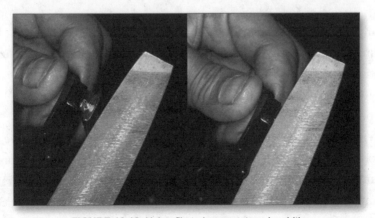

FIGURE 18.18: Using file to increase temple width

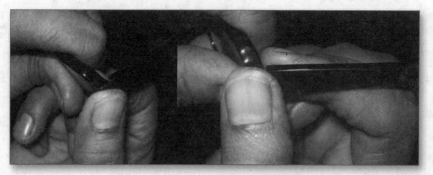

FIGURE 18.19: Using heat around the endpiece to reduce and increase temple width

FIGURE 18.20: Temple width and temple curve

that an inward curve of the temples around the ears is equally important to establish the parallel relation with the skull behind the ears. A body wear has to follow the body's contours to be comfortable in use. In order to provide temple curve for plastic frames apply heat to the section of the temple and run your thumb as shown in Figure 18.21 to curve the temples until you get your desired shape. For metal frames use double sides plastic-covered curve pliers. Do not use pliers with heated plastic frame. It will dent the frame.

TEMPLE BEND

In a hockey end temple frame (Fig. 18.22), the temple bend is an important fitting adjustment to ensure the frame stability on the wearer's face. The 3 sequential measurements that are critical while making

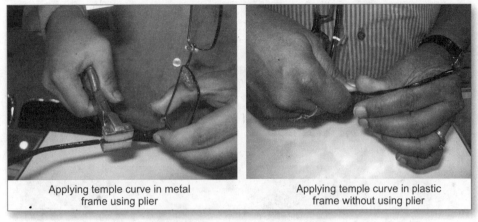

Applying temple curve in metal frame using plier

Applying temple curve in plastic frame without using plier

FIGURE 18.21: Applying temple curve

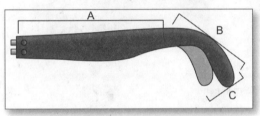

FIGURES 18.22 A to C: A. Length to the bend B. Length of the drop, C. Angle of the drop

adjustments for temple bend are shown in Flowchart 18.2.

Length to the bend is the distance between the back surfaces of the frame front to the midline of the bend. The distance between temple bend to the end of the temple is known as length of the drop. The temple bend so given form an angle between the length to bend and length of the drop which is known as angle of the drop. The angle of the drop is mostly 30°–45° when

a frame leaves the factory. The length to bend is measured in millimeter and usually ranges between 80–100 mm depending upon the frame size. Straight temple is usually measured from the back surface of the frame front to the extreme end.

Significance

Length to bend is probably the most noticed frame measurement. In hockey end temple it locks the frame from behind the ears and prevent slipping tendency.

Measuring Length to Bend

The millimeter ruler may be used to measure required length to bend for an individual from the spectacle plane to a point behind the top end of ears where the bone of the temporal skull start to turn inward.

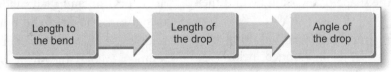

FLOWCHART 18.2: Different aspects of temple bend

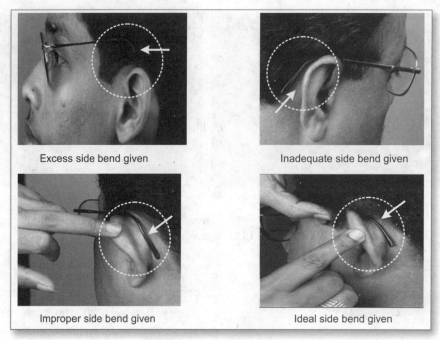

Excess side bend given

Inadequate side bend given

Improper side bend given

Ideal side bend given

FIGURE 18.23: Temple bends

Altering Temple Bend

An ideal, smooth and graceful temple bend should follow the following guideline as shown in Figure 18.23.

1. The length of the drop should not go below the lower part of the lobe of the ear.
2. The angle of the drop should not be very steep or very shallow.
3. The temple bend should begin immediately after passing over the top of the ear, and should have round and smooth bend so that it hugs the ears very gently.
4. The extreme end of the drop should follow the shape of the skull behind the ears.

The bend can be altered following the sequential steps as mentioned below as shown in Figure 18.24.

1. Apply heat at the point of existing bend and straighten out the temple end before creating a new bend. Do not try to change bend position without straightening the existing bend.
2. Now apply heat at a point where new bend is needed. Use your thumb or finger to create a new bend. Try to bend at the right point in the first try only. Repeated trying may develop wrinkles around the bend point and may not allow smooth and flowing bend.
3. Put the spectacle on wearer's face and check whether the temple bend wraps gently behind the ears. Correct the angle of drop and then modify inwards or outwards angle of end portion of the temples so that the end portion of the temples follows the shape of the bone behind the ears.

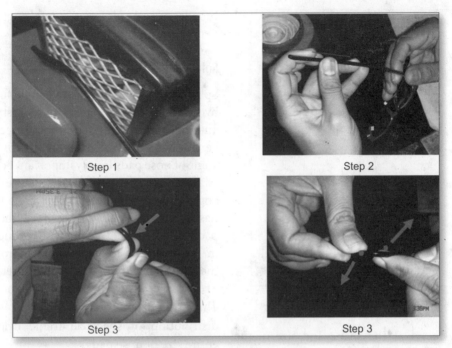

Step 1

Step 2

Step 3

Step 3

FIGURE 18.24: Altering side bend

4. In case of metal frame the end plastic tips can be removed and the temples may be cut and re-jacked when the drop is larger.

5. The ends of the cable curl sides have to be shaped to follow the anatomical form of the back of ear. Since they are spring, they can weaken over time and can also break.

NOSE PADS FITTING ADJUSTMENTS

Nose pads are the only parts of the metal frame front that touch the wearer's face. Nose pads are fined tuned for:
- Frontal angle
- Splay angle
- Vertical angle.

Frontal Angle

The frontal angle also known as spread angle represents the distance between 2 pads, i.e.

how far apart the pads are. The frontal angle is best observed from the front. It can be better explained with the help of a triangle. The 2 pads may be taken as the 2 sides of the triangle, when projected from the front of the face. The apex of the triangle lies on the forehead and the base of the triangle across the tip of the nose. The triangle so imagined may be divided into 2 equal halves by drawing an imaginary vertical line from the center of the forehead to the center of the tip of the nose. The angle with which each sides deviates from the vertical is called frontal angle as shown in Figure 18.25.

It is important to understand that the pads will lie on the sides of the nose only if the distance between the 2 pads is adequate. If the bridge of the frame is too wide, the frame will rest low on the nose and the line of sight will be close to the upper rim

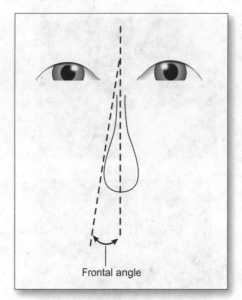

FIGURE 18.25: Frontal angle of nose pads

and vice versa. The shape and size of the nose influence the frontal angle of nose pads. People with concave and straight nose may need small frontal angle, whereas people with snub and flat nose may need larger frontal angle. In general, people with broader nose needs larger frontal angle than people with thinner nose.

Splay Angle

Splay angle of the nose is the angle formed by the side of the nose with a straight anteroposterior surface that bisects it vertically as shown in Figure 18.26. Splay angle of nose pads is very important because of variations in the shape of the nose. Splay angle should complement the angle of the nasal flanks at the point of contact. The nose pads need to be splayed out with the increase in the width of the nose as it approaches the inner corners of the eyes. Flatter nose needs larger splay angle than straight nose. This is important to ensure uniform weight distribution of spectacle frame over the entire size of nose pads.

The splay angle is viewed while looking through the spectacles frame. People with concave and straight nose may need small splay angle, whereas people with snub and flat nose may need larger splay angle. In

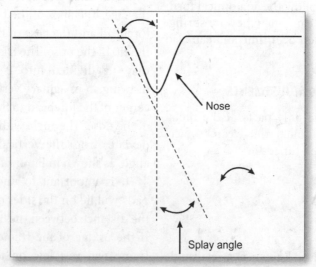

FIGURE 18.26: Splay angle

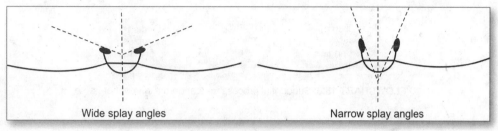

Wide splay angles

Narrow splay angles

FIGURE 18.27: Varying splay angles

general, people with flatter nose need larger splay angle than people with straight nose as shown in Figure 18.27.

Vertical Angle

The vertical angle of nose pads as seen from the sides of the face requires that the bottom edges of the pads is closer to the eyewires than the top edges of the pads as shown in Figure 18.28. The vertical angle of pads should always follow gravity. The vertical angle is controlled by the size of the loop of the pad arm and it determines the vertex distance of the front of the frame. Smaller loop of pad arm allows the vertex distance to minimum, whereas larger loop of pad arm allows keeping the front of the frame away from the cheeks by changing the vertical angle. A change in the pantoscopic angle is always followed by readjustments of vertical angle.

If all 3 angles are sitting flush with the skin, you have achieved a proper fit and the patient will be comfortable.

STANDARD ALIGNMENT

Finally spectacle frame is fine tuned for alignment. A number of adjustments are done that form the part of standard alignment. All adjustments for standard alignment are independent of face type and are critical for each frame and every wearer.

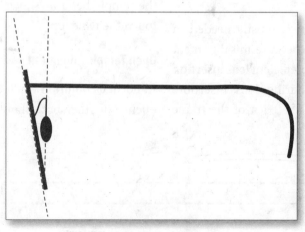

FIGURE 18.28: Vertical angle of nose pads

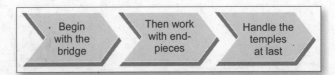

FLOWCHART 18.3: Sequential process for standard alignment of frame

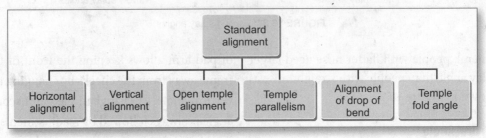

FLOWCHART 18.4: Different types of frame alignment adjustments

The ideal sequential process for standard alignment is shown in Flowchart 18.3.

The sequential process is important to eliminate repeated realignments as changes made in one portion will affect another portion of the frame. There are 6 different types of alignment adjustments that are critical in all frames. They are shown in Flowchart 18.4.

Horizontal Alignment

Horizontal alignment is mostly needed in case of plastic frame because misalignment occurs either due to inefficient lens insertion or skewed bridge during lens insertion. Put the ruler across the back of the frame front at the top of the pads and make sure that the endpieces are equidistant from the straight ruler when it is so aligned as shown in Figure 18.29.

Vertical Alignment

"4 point touch" is the most common test applied for vertical alignment. Put the open temple frame on the table top and make sure that 4 points—2 at the top eyewire and 2 at the temple bend as shown in Figure 18.30 touch the table top.

Open Temple Alignment

In normal condition when the 2 temples are opened out then both should make an angle

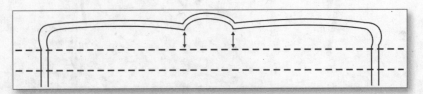

FIGURE 18.29: Frame front alignment

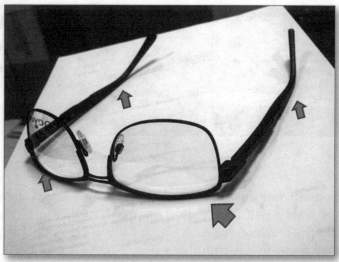

FIGURE 18.30: Four point touch

of 90°–95° with the front of the frame as shown in Figure 18.31.

Temple Parallelism

The relative angles of the temples to the frame front as seen from the sides determine the temple parallelism. In other words, pantoscopic angle of both the temples should be symmetrical. Put the frame upside down on a flat surface with temples open as shown in Figure 18.32 and note that both temples touch the flat surface. If both the temples are not touching the flat surface, they are misaligned. In case you find it difficult to note, gently touch one of the temples and check whether the frame sits solidly or wobbles. If it wobbles, it needs correction.

Alignment of Drop of Bend

A good standard alignment of drop of bend is one in which the ends of both temples are bent down equally as viewed from side. There are 2 checks to be done—check the equality of drop and check for equality of inward bending.

Temple Fold Angle

The last alignment adjustment is to fold the frame temples to closed position and observe the angle formed as the temples cross. The temples should fold so that they are parallel

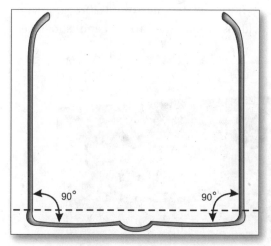

FIGURE 18.31: Open temple alignment

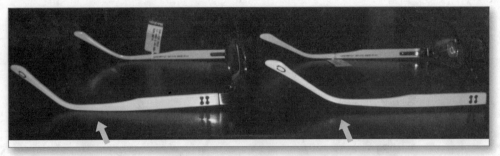

FIGURE 18.32: Temple parallelism

to one another as shown in Figure 18.33 or form slight angles from parallelism. Both the temples should cross each other exactly in the center of the frame in line with the center of the bridge.

SPECTACLE FRAME FITTING ASSESSMENT

A well-fit frame will come into physical contact with the wearer's face only at 3 points:

- The bridge of the nose
- On each side of the head including behind each ear.

If these 3 points are joined together it will form a triangle known as the 'fitting triangle' as shown in Figure 18.34.

A good spectacle frame fitting is an art that needs powerful and effective observation on the wearer's face. Observation, if done effectively following the well-defined sequential steps, will result in achieving the desired objectives. A fine sense of touch is an attribute of a good dispensing and you need to remember that you are fitting the spectacle frame for an individual for his comfort, not for just pretty look. Every individual has different facial anomalies. There are number of variations that can be seen as far as the shape of human skull is concerned. However, there is one unique aspect that is being observed commonly in most people, i.e. the anterior part of the head is wedge-shaped. The plane of the face is normally the narrowest that gradually widens around the earpoint and is followed

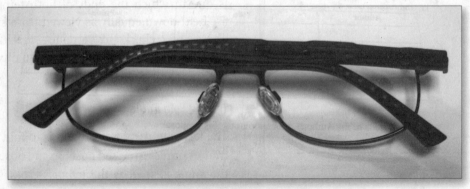

FIGURE 18.33: Temple fold angle

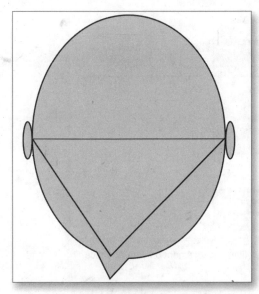

FIGURE 18.34: Fitting traingle

by another wedge-shaped part of the skull that points away from the face.

2 things are very important while fitting a spectacle frame with front and sides on a wedge shape head that determine the overall comfort. They are:

- Horizontal angle of sides
- Vertical angle of sides.

Horizontal angle of sides determines the position of spectacle frame on the wearer's face in horizontal plane. It relates to the angle of the fully opened temples that are being made with the plane of the spectacle frame front. Temple width and Frontal bow are 2 important fitting measurements that determine the fitting of spectacle frame in horizontal plane. Vertical angle of sides is the angle that the superior rim of the frame front makes with the temples of the frame near the joint area and is most commonly known as the pantoscopic angle.

It determines the frame alignment in the up and down position so that the front of the frame makes a parallel relation with the plane of the face. Thus, horizontal and vertical angle both together determine the position of front of the spectacle frame on the wearer's face. Once the correct position of the frame front is set, look at the fitting of temples. In hockey end temple the temple bend locks the frame from behind the ears and prevents dislocation of frame. There are 3 fitting adjustments to note—length to the bend, length of the drop and angle of the drop. It is usually believed that the length to the bend and angle of the drop holds the eyewear in place. Actually, it is the tangential relation of temples to skull behind the ears that holds the frame in place. At last, fix up the nose pads for metal frames. 2 nose pads hold the metal frame up off the nose and away from the face and assume the overall weight of the spectacle frame. Fine tuning the position of nose pads determines how comfortable the spectacle frame would be on the wearer's face. Nose pads position is fine tuned for frontal angle, splay angle and vertical angle of nose pads. Finally, take out the spectacle frame, put them on a flat surface with sides open and make sure that the spectacle frame maintains 4 point contacts and make' sure that the temples fold one over other before handling over the spectacle to the customer.

The summarization of sequential process of fitting assessment on wearer's face can be proposed as shown in Flowchart 18.5.

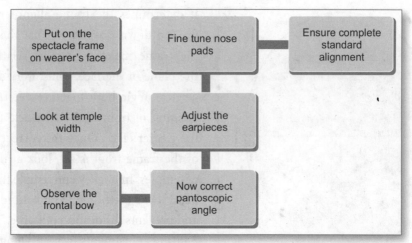

FLOWCHART 18.5: Sequential process of fitting assessment on wearer's face

POINTS TO REMEMBER

- Pantoscopic angle refers to the fitting alignment of spectacle frame front in its up and down position.
- Although retroscopic angle may be required on patient's with full cheeks, it is not a desirable condition.
- For every 2° of pantoscopic angle, the optical center for distance drops down by 1 mm.
- Pantoscopic angle in a frame may be increased by angling the temples downward from endpieces.
- When a spectacle frame leaves the factory, it always carry a certain degree of face form wrap which may vary from 5° to 7° from the frame front plane.
- Positive face form wrap brings the geometrical center of the frame nearer to the wearer's PD.
- When the measurement of patient's PD and GCD are identical, the frame should be adjusted with no face form.
- The temple width is the measure of the distance between the 2 temporal bones of the face at a level approximately 25–30 mm behind the spectacle plane, measured between the inner portions of one side to inner portion of other side.
- If the right temple of a frame is angled out, this will cause the right side of the frame front to move in.
- The distance between temple bend to the end of the temple is known as length of the drop.
- The frontal angle of the nose pads denotes the spread angle, i.e. how far apart the nose pads are.
- The vertical angle of nose pads is best seen from the sides of the face.
- The front of the frame may be raised by bringing the pad arms closer together.
- Angling the pad arms of a metal frame further apart will result in lowering the front.
- A well-fit frame will come into physical contact with the wearer at only 3 points— the bridge of the nose and on each side of the head including behind each ear.

DILEMMAS OF OPTICAL DISPENSING

Every time you cannot expect Mary Poppins to come dancing through your front door of your practice. There would be time when unexpected complaining patient may appear among the midst of merry throng and may proclaim in a voice that vibrates the entire atmosphere of your practice. Being a true professional, you have to handle the situation. You must be prepared to solve a variety of problems on daily basis, which occasionally defy logic and require the patience of highest degree combined with intelligent thinking. The objective of Chapter 19 is to provide the reader a guideline to handle multiple difficulties that appears on different occasions in an optical practice.

There are 3 parties to spectacle dispensing—patient, prescriber and dispensing optician (Flowchart 19.1).

There are times when the patient is unable to use the spectacle lenses comfortably. There may be several reasons—some of the reasons may be because of incompetences on the part of prescriber, some may be because of the dispensing optician, while others may be because of the patient himself.

Sometimes difficulties arise inherently because of the ocular conditions of the patient himself. For example, in higher degree of ametropia, even the best form lens

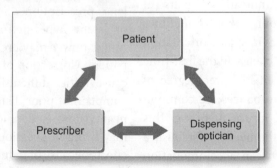

FLOWCHART 19.1: 3 parties involved in eyewear dispensing

does not entirely eliminate the disadvantage. Change in spatial perception and change in retinal image size are commonly associated difficulties with high degree of ametropia. Our perception of space is mediated by 2 mechanisms—one is based on perceptual judgment derived from past experience and the other is based on the stereoscopic effect derived because of the 2 eyes. Anomalous spatial perception is possible if there is any incongruity between 2 eyes. Magnification and minifications are common with high degree of ametropia also causes difficulties in spatial perception as magnified objects are perceived as closer and minified objects are perceived as lying at far distance. Besides, certain monochromatic aberrations are also induced which are more pronounced when seen through the lens periphery. They degrade and deshape the image quality when seen obliquely. Correction of anisometropia may be accompanied by muscle imbalance because the asymmetric spectacle lenses that are prescribed in an attempt to equalize visual acuity create their own asymmetric prismatic effects between the eyes which may result in both asthenopia and diplopia. Correction of astigmatism may lead to spatial disorientation. This nonuniform magnification or minification results in meridional aniseikonia that sometimes produces disturbances in spatial orientation and asthenopia, particularly in the first-time spectacle wearer. Even in lower degree of ametropia some disturbances are common on wearing spectacle for the first time. This may be because of the need to establish a new relationship between accommodation and convergence. The new wearer may feel

a short-lived pulling sensation of eye. The complicated process of vision needs motor coordination of 2 eyes and the sensory unification of their respective views of the object. Responding to brain orders, the external muscles act to coordinate the 2 eyes with each other and internal muscles bring the image into focus. The separation between 2 eyes brings in slight different perspective of the world that allows stereoscopic view. Thus the process of vision is highly balanced and controlled where efficient teaming of 2 eyes is needed. Anything that makes it difficult for the eyes to work together may cause dizziness, headache, or reading difficulties.

The prescriber may have carried out a poor refraction or have ordered a wrong prescription. Sometimes the prescriber may overlook small factors like patient's previous correction, importance of room lights during refraction, patient's expectations and patient's lifestyle and profession before writing the prescription. In most cases it may not create difficulties, but in some cases overlooking these small factors may prove fatal. A sudden prescription of high correction to a patient who has never worn any correction may not be tolerant to him or the patient may not find it comfortable to accept great change in his lens prescription. Sometimes correction of latent hypermetropia or reduction of minus power may create difficulties for the patient. Correction of latent hyperopia may cause initial difficulties. Most patient will complain of poor distance vision and good near vision. Reducing minus prescription may bring in occasional unpleasant optical effects because of reduced vision quality and change in the need for convergence. One of the most common faults is to prescribe too strong addition for reading in patient with presbyopia, as no rule can be laid down for presbyopic prescription.

The dispensing of spectacles may occasionally be at fault and responsible for intolerance. These may relate to frame selection or any other aspect of frame fitting. In practice, the form of the lens is often left to the lens manufacturer, but the optician should mention the need for any specific lens form in certain cases. The lens centering and degree of pantoscopic tilt also must be extremely accurate. There are certain frame shapes that may be unsuitable in the higher degree of ametropia. So far as the lenses are concerned, points of importance are occurrence of small change in the vertex distance in strong power lens, a change in base curve, a change from flat lens to meniscus form or toric form.

The limitations of optics also bring in difficulties as no lens is 100% perfect. All lenses degrade in their performance as you see away from its center. The best lens is one that is defined by peripheral area of moderate performance, intermediate area of good performance, and central area of best performance. Above all no lens can transmit 100% rays of light. Some of the light is lost because of absorption and surface reflection. Occasionally these small factors become points of great concern.

When a spectacle lens is worn, a series of changes is noticed in visual performance. Some of these changes are intended and others come along. A notable behavior change is seen in the wearer as plus lens wearer emphasizes more on ground because of expanded space horizon. On the contrary, a minus lens wearer emphasizes more on figure because of constricted space horizon. A plus lens wearer is peripherally more aware, whereas minus lens wearer finds himself good at central detailing. Plus lens brings in base in prismatic effect, whereas minus lens brings in base out prismatic effect. Neuromuscular mechanism of the ocular system is affected through their influence on accommodation. A young hyperope who could manage to see distance with accommodation and needed to accommodate more to see near, now does not need to make an effort to accommodate for distance vision. A young myope who could see near without using accommodation has to start accommodating to see at near.

Therefore, it is quite likely that sometimes a new spectacle correction can take quite some time before being comfortable to the user. This does not necessarily mean that glasses are wrong. As long as straight ahead vision is clear, most effects will resolve completely within a week or two. But for some patients it may be an unpleasant experience as they may experience certain unusual sensations. Some of the common unusual sensations may be one or more of the followings.

SIZE JUDGMENT

The universal truth is that plus lens makes the image larger and minus lens makes the image smaller. However, the effect of magnification or minification may be reduced by reducing the vertex distance of the spectacles, making them closer to eyes. Alterations in base curve may also alter this effect. Steepening the base curve of the lens may bring in a bit of magnification for myopes and flattening the base curve may minimize the effect of magnification for hyperopes.

DISTANCE JUDGMENT

Our brain carries a past experience of an object of regard. When we put on the new glasses, plus lens makes the object look bigger and minus lens makes the object look smaller. So when we look at an object with plus power, the brain wrongly decides that it must be closer. The opposite is true for myopes. Usually it goes after a few days. Myopes adapts quicker than hyperopes.

GIDDYNESS

Our visual system is connected to the vestibular system. The job of the vestibular system is to sense changes in motion. The vestibular system works in conjunction with the visual system to detect head and body motion as well as eye movement. When the plus lens magnifies the size of object, the equal vestibular response is not enough and eyes need to make a larger angular deviation to remain on track. This may cause motion sickness which leads to giddiness. This occurs because of disagreement between what eyes tell the brain and what ears tell the brain. Giddyness may also occur when one eye is less involved in the vision process than the other. This may be because of deterioration in vision or spatial awareness.

SLOPPING

A plus astigmatic lens magnifies more in one meridian than the other, whereas a minus astigmatic lens minifies more in one meridian than other. It means that retinal image of a circle will be oval instead of circle. A desk and floor may appear having sloped, door frames may appear distorted and a square paper may appear trapezoidal when there is great change in

cylinder or in axis of cylinder lens. This is a strange perception that lapses with time, but it is really disturbing. If it does not go over a period of time, it may be necessary to adjust the cylinder or the axis and with new correction the wearer may not see as clearly as with the previous correction.

FEELING TOO STRONG POWER

This is quite common when there is a major change or a new spectacle is worn for the first time. The brain takes time to adapt. You can apply a trick to manage. Ask the wearer to look at the distant object through the spectacle lens and pull the spectacle away from the eyes. In case of minus power, if it deteriorates the vision quality, it implies that the correction is optimum. If the vision remains same, it implies a slight reduction in minus power is justified. In case of plus power, pulling the spectacle away from eyes improves near vision with the optimum correction.

A patient with latent hypermetropia when corrected may also report the same. He may report good vision at near, but may complain of blurry distant vision. A short adaptation period would resolve the problem. Alternatively reduction in correction is warranted. In an extreme case change in lens index or lens curvature may also be the reason.

LIGHT SENSITIVITY

Sometimes due to incorrect positioning of optical center in its vertical direction, vertical phoria may be induced which may cause light sensitivity, difficulties with glare and reflection. Some patients when switched from tinted to clear lens may also complain of light sensitivity.

MILD HEADACHE

A change in prescription or vertical phoria may also lead to headache.

Intensity of new experience, consciousness about new glasses and lack of initial confidence and attitude to pinpoint the smallest defect in the glasses may contribute to headache.

HALOES AROUND LIGHT

Very rarely patient complains of haloes around the eyes which are specially noticed around car lights or tail lights at night. Usually this is not associated with optical lenses, more associated with ocular pathology. But patient notices this when they use the new lenses. They learn to live with the same.

HEAD MOTION SICKNESS

Head motion sickness occurs because of poor stabilization of retinal image during head motion in the horizontal plane. This is more pronounced if the spectacle frame shape is steep rectangular or the patient's IPD is very narrow. The optics of the lens says that as the line of gaze shifts from the center of the lens to the periphery and prismatic effect is induced. It is larger as the distance from the point to optical center increases. With low power these effects are rarely noticed.

FLOOR SEEMS CONCAVE

Many times after putting on new correction the patient feels as if he is standing in a bowl, or vertical objects seem taller than normal, or he feels as if he is walking uphill. These may be the symptoms of a hyperope looking above the optical center of a pair of glasses.

FLOOR SEEMS CONVEX

Sometimes the patient feels as if he is standing on a hilltop, or vertical objects seem shorter than normal, or he feels as if he is walking downhill. This may be the symptoms of a myope looking above optical center of minus lenses.

Most of the above situations can be overcome after a short adaptation period of time. The patient needs to understand that getting used to a new prescription or a new lens requires him to break his past visual habits. It is, therefore, important that the dispensing optician explains adaptation verbally before and after dispensing, and supply written instructions to reinforce the information. The better the patient understands what he needs to do to adjust, the better are the chances of successful adaptation. The patient may take 1–2 weeks to adapt or in some cases the adaptation period may stretch to even 3–4 weeks. Because we see with our brains, it takes a while for the eyes and the brain to coordinate getting used to a new prescription. The length of time for adaptation depends on:

- The strength of the prescription.
- Whether there has been a significant change in prescription.
- Whether you are wearing glasses for the first time.
- Or you have gone from a large frame to a smaller frame or vice versa.
- Or from contact lenses to glasses, there may be a longer adjustment period.
- The same applies for adjusting to bifocals, specially no-line bifocals.

During the period of adaptation the patient may have a bit of discomfort, but eventually the glasses should become very comfortable. If you have glasses for the first time, the best way to get used to them is to wear them as often as possible. Using only intermittently will only delay the adaptation. There are certain times when the patient cannot adapt to the lenses even after 3–4 weeks. Under such a situation the patient needs to be referred back to the concerned optometrist.

POINTS TO REMEMBER

- High power lenses change the size of the retinal image. Plus lens magnifies and minus lens minimizes.

- Spectacle lens corrects the refractive error and at the same time induces the aberrations when seen through the lens periphery.
- Square paper looks trapezoidal is a common complain when there is great change in cylinder or in axis of cylinder lens.
- A patient with latent hypermetropia may complain good vision at near, but distant vision may be blurry.
- Incorrect placement of optical center in its vertical direction may lead to vertical phoria that may induce light sensitivity.

CASE STUDIES

The real world is always more engaging than theory and learning from real life experiences is more effective. Chapter 20 is set to talk about various real life experiences that I could gather while dealing with my patients for their spectacle dispensing. Although I could see thousands of cases, I collected only a few to provide the real life feel of spectacle dispensing to the readers.

CASE 1

A presbyopic male, age 65 years, whose lens prescription showed:

RE –3.50 Dsph / –1.25 Dcyl @80 6/9
LE –4.00 Dsph / –1.00 Dcyl @100 6/9
BE Near Add +2.25 Dsph
Frame type: Plastic full rim frame
Lens type: Progressive addition lens
Complain: Vision clarity is poor in reading

Initial Thoughts

Initially when I attended the patient, I thought it could be because of near addition.

An immediate thought that came to mind, "Probably there was a need for little higher near addition".

Re-examination

1. Temporary ink markings of progressive addition lenses were restored.
2. Checked the lens power using lensometer.
3. All frame fittings were checked and compared with previous spectacle.
4. Fitting cross position was checked again.
5. Refraction was done again and it was found that the lens prescription was satisfactory and the patient is not very sensitive to changes in near addition between +2.25 Dsph and +2.50 Dsph. But +2.75 Dsph near addition was not acceptable to him. However, lifting the near zone little up indicated little improvement in reading, but the patient's comments "not as good as previous spectacle" was very critical. It was a great clue to proceed.

Past Habits

- *Lens prescription*: Not much change in lens power.
- *Past lens type*: Univis D bifocal.
- *Past frame type*: Large size and square shape plastic frame with segment height placed at lower lid margin.

Proposed Solution

Based upon the results of re-refraction and his past experience of Univis D bifocal, I decided to change the lens type to Univis D bifocal in the same frame with same prescription.

Result

Patient reported immediate sense of comfort with a soft smile that was full of contentment.

Impression

Past habits are very important specially in case of matured presbyope. Lens selection should never be done with predecided approach. You need to discover the need for the change and then you need to establish it to his lifestyle so that the patient himself tries to adapt to changes. At the age of 65 years we cannot expect a patient to adapt to a new type of lens design as he may not be motivated because of lack of need.

CASE 2

A male, age 73 years, whose lens prescription showed:
RE +1.25 Dcyl @180 6/18
LE +1.25 Dsph / +0.75 Dcyl @180 6/18
BE Add + 2.50 Dsph   N6

Frame type: Full rim metal frame
Lens type: Executive bifocal in clear crown glass
Complaint: When he tilts his spectacle down to one side on the face, things look straight, otherwise things look tilted

Initial Thoughts

Initially when I attended the patient, I thought the problem could be because of cylinder axis. So I thought to relook at the refraction specially for cylinder axis. I proceeded with this thought in mind.

Re-examination

1. Checked the lens power using lensometer.
2. All frame fittings were checked and compared with previous spectacle. The frame size difference was observed. Previous frame was larger than the new frame.
3. Refraction was done again and it was found that there was no change in lens prescription and the wearer was not very sensitive to changes in axis and power.

Past Habits

- *Lens prescription*:
  RE +1.00 Dcyl @ 09
  LE +1.00 Dsph /+0.50 Dcyl @ 179
  Add +2.00 Dsph.
- *Past lens type*: Photochromatic glass Executive bifocal.
- *Past frame type*: Large size and square shape plastic full rim frame with large B measurement. The segment height was observed to be lower than lower lid.

Proposed Solution

It was decided to make a new spectacle with following changes:

- *Lens prescription*:
  RE +1.25 Dcyl @180
  LE +1.00 Dsph / +0.75 Dcyl @180
  Add +2.50 Dsph
- *Lens type*: Executive bifocal in clear crown glass.
- *Frame type*: The significant difference noted was only in the frame size because of which the segment height was also lowered than the same in the new frame. It prompted me to try changing frame to larger size with little lower segment height.

Result

It worked and the patient reported immediate relief.

Impression

Sometimes it is difficult to justify the reason for your action while managing patient's complaining for nonadaptation of spectacle. Patient's symptoms may not be relevant. Or, it is also quite likely that patient is unable to communicate you the exact difficulties that he is facing. If logical thinking does not work, go by lateral thinking and if both does not work you may proceed by your gut feeling or previous experiences. Complain management is all about being thorough in your approach. It needs careful listening and powerful observation on every little aspect of spectacle dispensing.

CASE 3

A male, age 46 years, whose lens prescription showed:
RE −2.00 Dsph / −3.25 Dcyl @170
LE −1.25 Dsph/ −1.50 Dcyl @50
BE Add +1.75 Dsph
Frame type: Full rim metal frame
Lens type: CR 39 progressive with ARC
Complaint: When he looks through the corner of the lens, he sees more clearly than when he sees through the center of the lens

Initial Thoughts

It was unusual complain. Usually with any progressive lens temporal corner carries unwanted astigmatism and prismatic effect that affect the visual performance adversely.

Re-examination

1. Temporary ink markings of progressive addition lenses were restored and their standard position was checked to ensure that right lens is not fitted in left eyewire.
2. Checked the lens power using lensometer.
3. Fitting cross position was checked again.
4. The patient did not find any improvement even after modifying frame fitting for frontal bow and pantoscopic tilt.
5. Refraction was not done again as the patient was already using another spectacle comfortably with the same prescription.

Past Habits

- *Lens prescription*: No change was seen in lens prescription when compared with the old lenses.

- *Past lens type*: CR 39 Univis D bifocal lens
- *Past frame type*: The patient had several spectacles and all being different styles.

Proposed Solution

It was decided to change the lens type with Univis D bifocal lens.

Result

The wearer reported immediate relief.

Impression

While dealing with the complaining patients, there are times when it is possible that what the patient is stating may not be what he intends to say. He may not have correct words to explain the nature of his difficulties. As a professional optician it is your responsibility to try and drag out the root cause of his dissatisfaction. Under such situations never cut off by saying "yes, I understand" or "no, you are wrong." Listen patiently and put a thought on all that he says. Finally, follow the course that restores the patient's satisfaction.

CASE 4

A male, age 55 years, whose lens prescription showed:
   RE −3.00 Dsph /−1.00 Dcyl @ 90
   LE −2.00 Dsph /−0.50 Dcyl @90
   BE Near Add +2.50 Dsph
Frame type: Full rim plastic frame
Lens type: CR 39 progressive addition lens
Complaint: He has to lift his spectacle up, to read and vision on either side is not comfortable. Overall he was not very happy with spectacle lens

Initial Thoughts

It was a general complain of all first time user of progressive lenses specially when a matured presbyopic patient uses progressive addition lens for the first time. Initially I thought that it could be probably because of either poor counseling or incomplete understanding of the patient about the application of progressive addition lenses. As far as reading difficulty is concerned I thought selection of corridor length might have been longer. Based on these thoughts I adjusted the nose pads and explained him about the anatomy of the progressive addition lens and advised him to use it for some days. After a few days he came back with the same complain.

Re-examination

1. Temporary ink markings of progressive addition lenses were restored and all relevant checks were done.
2. Checked the lens power using lensometer.
3. Re-examination of refractive error was done and was found to be perfect.

Past Habits

- *Lens prescription*: The lens prescription was not an issue as there was no significant difference.
- *Past lens type*: His previous spectacle had E-style bifocal lenses. For the new spectacle he himself opted for progressive addition lenses because he had seen his friends working happily on computer with progressive addition lens. He developed his own conception about the progressive addition lens and was not ready to change his opinion.

- *Occupations*: Working on computers for more than 6–8 hours for data feeding from text document kept at the sides.
- *Past frame type*: Plastic frame.

Proposed Solution

Since, there was no issue with distance vision, I proposed him to change the lens type, he did not accept at all as he was too keen to use progressive lenses. I was left with no option but to look for some factor on which I could talk to him and I found the difference in frame type and its placement on his face. The vertex distance noted was little more, hence I advised him to transfer the lens into some metal frame with nose pads to which he agreed. The lens was transferred and given to him. While giving the new frame I explained him complete anatomy of progressive addition lens and adaption needed for the same. I also gave him fair deal of idea about his occupation and need for occupational progressive lenses. In order to re-establish his lost confidence, I gave him my business card and assure all possible after care.

Some 3 days later he came back saying progressive lens was not working for him and requested to change. By now he accepted the limitations of progressive lenses. I made 2 spectacles for him—one spectacle with E-style bifocal lens that had lens prescription for distance and near, another spectacle with E-style bifocal lens having lens power for intermediate and near distance.

Result

He was given a desktop and asked to notice the difference. An immediate sense of relief was seen on his face.

Impression

Understanding customer's psychology and keeping patience is the key to successful management of dissatisfied patients. While lifestyle and occupational questioning, it is important that you dig deeper. A computer user can be benefited by progressive addition lenses, but a data feeder who needs to move his eyes and head a lot would be benefitted either by occupational lens or specially design lens for the occupation. While dealing with the patient I also learnt that a self-motivated customer for progressive lens is not ready to listen against progressive lens as he has seen his close friends using the same comfortably. He takes time to break his opinion to accept your advice. I also learnt the importance of educating the customer and realized the fact that there is a big difference between informed customer and educated customer. If you do not educate the customer, he collects information from any available sources and that might register in his mind.

CASE 5

A presbyopic male, age 58 years, whose lens prescription showed:
  RE +1.50 Dsph 6/6
  LE +1.25 Dsph 6/6
  BE Near Add +2.75 Dsph
Frame type: Metal supra frame
Lens type: Progressive addition lens
Complain: Feeling strain while reading and overall the spectacle lens was not comfortable

Initial Thoughts

My first impression was it could be because of fitting of spectacle on his face as the spectacle frame showed insufficient pantoscopic tilt on his face. I tried several changes in the frame fitting but the improvement was not satisfactory.

Re-examination

1. Temporary ink markings of progressive addition lenses were restored and all relevant checks were done.
2. Checked the lens power using lensometer.
3. *Lens prescription*: It was found that the lens prescription was satisfactory and there was a small change in the near addition only from +2.50 Dsph to +2.75 Dsph. However, lifting the near spectacle lens little up indicated little improvement in reading, but the patient's comments "not as good as previous spectacle" was very critical.
4. His primary occupational visual need was for reading.

Past Habits

- *Lens prescription*: No significant change in lens power.
- *Past lens type*: Progressive addition lens.
- *Past frame type*: Little smaller in size than new full rim metal frame.

Proposed Solution

While assessing the lens fit I noticed that the line of sight does not pass through the center of the near power circle during reading which looked like little out. Eventually I measured the distance between 2 fitting cross; it did not match with the measured monocular distance PD of the patient. I decided to change the frame to smaller size frame so that I can alter fitting cross position. The whole idea was to save the lens cost and restore the patient's satisfaction. Fortunately the patient agreed to change to smaller size. The lens was re-edged to fit the new frame and fitting cross placement was corrected.

Result

This worked wonderfully, patient went back with huge satisfaction on his face.

Impression

A methodical approach with diligent thinking gives rise to a process where one correct step paves the way for another correct step and ultimately leads you to find out the solution. I changed the frame fitting, it did not work; I checked the lens power, found it perfect; and finally I restored the progressive marking and got the solution. Sometimes complaining patient provides clues that can be used find to the solution.

CASE 6

A presbyopic male, age 54 years, whose lens prescription showed:
RE −9.00 Dsph 6/6
LE −9.50 Dsph 6/6
BE Near Add +2.50 Dsph
Frame type: Metal full rim frame
Lens type: Mineral glass photochromatic Univis D bifocal lens
Complain: Black spots are seen in the field of vision for a moment. When he moves his head they disappear suddenly

Initial Thoughts

The immediate thought that came to mind to advise a dilated eye examination to rule out the possibility of floaters in the vitreous.

Re-examination

Dilated eye examination report indicated that there were no floaters in vitreous and retina was absolutely healthy. The examining eye doctor categorically pointed out that his eyes were absolutely healthy and there was no change in the lens prescription also and advised to keep a note on the symptoms to visit again if problem persists. It is quite likely that sometimes a problem may not be detected at the initial stage.

Past Habits

- *Lens prescription*: Not much change in lens power.
- *Past lens type*: Univis D bifocal.
- *Past frame type*: Metal full rim frame.

Proposed Solution

I decided to continue with the same lenses to which the patient agreed.

Result

Patient went back with a sense of contentment for having got utmost after care and good advice.

Impression

Most patients are very apprehensive about the performance of their new lenses when they make their new spectacle. In the process they check the lens performance in various ways and if they notice any unusual sensation or perception or feeling they attribute the reason to their new lenses. This is a difficult situation to manage because they firmly believe that the new problem is because of new lenses.

Sometimes it is also possible that what the patient is saying may not be what he intends to say. He may be in a process where he is trying to rule out different probabilities. As a professional optician, you must be prepared to solve a variety of problems on daily basis that may occasionally defy logic and require patience.

CASE 7

A presbyopic male, age 46 years, whose lens prescription showed:
RE Plano 6/6
LE –1.00 Dcyl @90 6/6
BE Near Add +2.00 Dsph
Frame type: Metal full rim frame
Lens type: Progressive addition lens
Complain: Vision disturbances with progressive lens

Initial Thoughts

The complaining patient was a regular old patient who had always been making his spectacle from us and it was for the first time that he had any complain. My past experience with the patient was also very positive. He had always been speaking short, precise and straight. He never appreciated too much sales driven communication and whenever anything went against his likings, he had been very harsh. Overall he was a calm and composed person. Probably because of these reasons I also did not expect any cooperation from him. Since the complain was little vague I decided to ensure that I must spend some time with him to perform all tests and checks silently in front of him. With this initial thought I proceeded.

Re-examination:

1. Temporary ink markings of progressive addition lenses were restored and all relevant checks were done.
2. Checked the lens power using lensometer.
3. It was found that the lens prescription was satisfactory and he was not accepting any change in lens prescription. However, when I started modifying fitting adjustments of spectacle frame, he noticed improvement. He took the spectacle and suddenly got up to move out.

Past Habits

- *Lens prescription*: Not much change in lens power. Distance lens prescription was same and near addition increased from +1.50 Dsph to +2.00 Dsph.
- *Past lens type*: Progressive addition lenses.
- *Past frame type*: Always using classic style regular plastic or metal frames.
- *Past experience*: Happy user of progressive addition lenses.

Proposed Solution

The patient himself found the solution while modifying the frame fitting adjustments on his face. I tried to ask him whether he was happy or not, but as expected no reply came from him. We both went out of the clinic together. While we did so the new spectacle was on his eyes.

Result

Here it is difficult for me to exactly mention whether he was satisfied or not, but he got up and went out of the clinic with me and started talking to me about prevailing promotional offer that he noticed seeing the posters and table tops displayed in the store. I conveyed him very gently that we were having huge discount offers on frames. In reply he asked me to show him some frames that were available on discounts. He did not take lot of time, selected one frame and asked me to pack the frame only.

Impression

There were 2 reasons why I did not try and sell him lenses:

1. He came because of some difficulties with his spectacle and not to buy anything.
2. His dissatisfaction was for lens performance and not for frame.
3. The impression of his personality in my mind.

Had I insisted upon lenses, he might not have taken the frame or he might have been annoyed with me. Under any of above circumstances I might have lost the opportunity to sell the frame. In sales, there are times when you need to refrain from being aggressive.

CASE 8

A presbyopic female, age 54 years, whose lens prescription showed:
  RE +1.50 Dsph / +0.75 Dcyl @ 80 6/6
  LE +1.25 Dsph / +0.25 Dcyl @100 6/6
  BE Near Add +2.25 Dsph
Frame type: Metal full rim frame
Lens type: Progressive addition lens

> *Complain*: Strange visual discomfort with new lenses and she restated that her previous spectacle was better than new one

Initial Thoughts

It was an exaggerated complaint. Immediately I thought that the patient had not tried the spectacle for sufficient period of time or she must have put on the spectacle and when found little uncomfortable she must have kept it aside. With these initial thoughts I asked her whether she used the spectacle or not to which she confirmed that she did not use it for more than a few minutes.

Re-examination

1. Temporary ink markings of progressive addition lenses were restored and all relevant checks were done.
2. Checked the lens power using lensometer.
3. It was found that the lens prescription was absolutely correct. There was no need to change lens prescription. When I checked the spectacle fitting on her face I found that it was not at all adjusted to her face. I asked whether she came personally to collect the spectacle or not. As expected again she told me that she did not come personally to collect the spectacle.

Past Habits

- *Lens prescription*:
  RE +2.00 Dsph / +1.00 Dcyl @ 80 6/6
  LE +1.75 Dsph / +0.25 Dcyl @100 6/6
  BE Near Add +2.00 Dsph.
- *Past lens type*: Progressive addition lenses.

- *Past frame type*: She used varieties of style of frame in the past and always buying a new style frame.
- *Past experience*: Happy user of progressive addition lenses.

Proposed Solution

I made the complete fitting adjustments on her face so that the spectacle frame fit her snugly and is stable at the desired place. She noticed lot of improvement and went back with satisfaction.

Result

Next day I talked to the patient over phone and enquired about her satisfaction. She replied that it was perfect.

Impression

Patience is the key to success while dealing with such patients. Most often they amplify their complains and present them in such a manner as if the spectacle made is absolutely wrong or intolerable. They feel that they will put on their new spectacle and everything will be absolutely clear. Over a period of time I have experienced that patients who amplify their difficulties are typically self-conceited type. I may be incorrect while mentioning but I have my own experience and I have noticed that they carry an inflated self-image. They always want more attention and like others to dance to their tune. Probably because they are highly pampered and their all whims and fancies have been catered.

CASE 9

A presbyopic female, age 50 years, whose lens prescription showed:
RE Plano
LE –3.00 Dsph / –1.00 Dcyl @180
BE Near Add +2.25 Dsph
Frame type: Metal full rim frame
Lens type: Progressive addition lens
Complain: Difficulty in seeing on wider horizon, I can see anywhere with my previous lenses, but with the new one I find difficulties even with little eye movement

Initial Thoughts

The patient was a happy user of progressive lenses since long. He had another spectacle with same prescription with which he had no difficulties. As he told me his difficulties the first thing that came to my mind was to check the fitting cross position. With these initial thoughts I asked him whether he had similar difficulties with his other glasses or not to which he confirmed that he had been using it without any difficulties since long.

Re-examination

1. Temporary ink markings of progressive addition lenses were restored and all relevant checks were done.
2. Checked the lens power using lensometer.
3. It was found that the fitting cross position was incorrect. In right eye it was little out and in left eye it was little in.

Past Habits

- *Lens prescription*: No change, using similar lens prescription.

- *Past lens type*: Progressive addition lenses.
- *Past frame type*: Full rim metal frame.

Proposed Solution

I tried to modify horizontal inclination of frame front to check whether any improvement is possible or not, but the effort was in vain. I also tried to shift the spectacle frame front to one side, the patient reported little improvement. It was just an effort to be sure whether the fitting cross position is creating difficulties or not. I remarked the new fitting cross position and made the new lenses. He reported satisfaction.

Result

Next day I talked to the patient over phone and enquired about his satisfaction. He replied that it was perfect.

Impression

Optical dispensing is based on basic established guideline. Overlooking those guideline will always lead to patient dissatisfaction. The thumb rule for progressive addition lens dispensing is aligning the fitting cross with the monocular pupillary distance of the wearer as fitting cross represents the alignment point of the lens design. While fitting, it is located at the center of the pupil in straight ahead gaze. If there is any mismatch, the line of sight will not pass through the center of the viewing zone, thereby creating difficulties in binocular viewing zone sizes. This is very critical in progressive addition lenses as the width of usable zone of clear vision is significantly reduced.

CASE 10

A presbyopic female, age 54 years, whose lens prescription showed:
RE –9.25 Dsph / –1.75 Dcyl @30 6/9
LE –9.25 Dsph / –1.50 Dcyl @140 6/9
BE Near Add +1.50 Dsph
Frame type: Metal full rim frame
Lens type: Progressive addition lens
Complain: While reading vision is not comfortable, cannot keep the spectacle for longer time on eyes. I feel as if somebody is pulling my eyes.

Initial Thoughts

The complaining patient was a very old patient who had always been making her spectacle from us and it was for the first time that she had any complain in last so many years. She had been carrying enormous amount of trust in me as because sometimes back she was referred to me by one of my very happy patient.

Initially when she complained me, I modified face form wrap and ensured that the spectacle frame fit her snugly on her face. She told me that it seemed to be better than before. Based upon her response I asked her to use it for some days in the expectation to improve further. 2 days later she came back and reported that she could not wear it even for an hour or so. Immediately, I thought to recheck refraction.

Re-examination

1. When she came for the first time all temporary ink markings of progressive addition lenses were restored and all relevant checks were done to ensure that there is no mistake in lens dispensing. I also checked the lens power using lensometer and modified the new spectacle frame fitting in accordance with her previous spectacle frame.

2. On her second visit when she again complained the same difficulties, I re-refracted to ensure that the lens prescription given was correct. It was found that she was not very sensitive to change in power. She reported the near equal response when I compared her previous lens prescription with the new one.

Past Habits

- *Lens prescription*:
  RE –9.00 Dsph / –1.75 Dcyl @30 6/9
  LE –9.00 Dsph / –1.25 Dcyl @140 6/9
  BE Near Add +1.50 Dsph.
- *Past lens type*: Progressive addition lenses.
- *Past frame type*: Always using classic style regular plastic or metal frames.
- *Past experience*: Happy user of progressive addition lenses.

Proposed Solution

The new lens prescription was made as:
RE –9.00 Dsph / –2.00 Dcyl @35 6/9
LE –9.00 Dsph / –1.25 Dcyl @145 6/9
BE Near Add +1.75 Dsph.

The new lenses were made and when she came to take delivery of the new lenses, I gave her enough time to feel the difficulties, but she reported immediate satisfaction. She took the spectacle and told that she would be able to tell only after using the same for a day.

Result

2 days later when I gave her call to enquire, she reported that the new spectacle was perfect and she was happy.

Impression

There were reasons why I did not try and reverify the prescription when she came first. The change in prescription was not significant; therefore, I wanted to save the cost of replacing the lens. Moreover, the amount of care and concern that I showed also influenced her positively and was multiplied manifold because of positive credibility that she was carrying about my sincerity because of her past experience.

Had she insisted, probably I would have done everything in her first visit only.

In practice sometimes you need to look at the opportunity to save losses.

However, when she came again with same complain I immediately took her to clinic to verify the lens prescription because myopes are always very sensitive to change in lens prescription. Unless the change is warranted, small changes should always be avoided as I did in this case. The change in lens prescription may bring in unpleasant optical effects because of the need to establish new accommodation—convergence relation.

TIPS TO HANDLE PATIENT'S COMPLAINS

1. Be concerned, positive and apologetic while handling patient complains.
2. Let the patient speak out all his grievances. While he is speaking do not interrupt by saying "yes I understand". Or do not try and prove him wrong.
3. Listen and let your eyes speak that you are listening.
4. Put a thought on all points that he communicates and also on what he should have pointed out but could not do so.
5. Complete all checks and tests needed to verify the accuracy of lens power and other measurements.
6. Compare with the past habits with respect to lens power, frame type, frame fitting, lens type and take a note of any changes.
7. Try and modify frame fitting on the face and see if there is any improvement.
8. Try and establish the cause of the difficulties. It may not be possible all the time but in case it is possible it can be a great help.
9. If needed, ask your optometrists to re-refract.
10. If the point is reached where no care, concern, and compassion will resolve the situation, give the complete refund. Give an emotional end to the instance and emotional reason for the patient to come back.

Complain handling for nonadaptation of the spectacle should begin following the formula of LAST where "L" stands for listening the patient very carefully and patiently, "A" stands for being apologetic to the patient for inconvenience caused, "S" stands for satisfying the patient with remedial correction and "T" stands for thanking the patient for putting up the complain and patient cooperation. Listening is probably the most important element of complain handling in optical dispensing. Unless the patient speaks out his difficulties, it is not possible to find out the remedial solution. Apply the formula of "Triple L" that entails that the dispensing optician must listen, listen and listen while handling the complaining patient. The first listen stands for him to listen patiently all the grievances of the patient. Since the patient has difficulties, he is probably upset, so do not interrupt when he starts saying. The second listen for him is to relay the nature of his problem. Unless he speaks out his problem completely, the optician cannot even think out the way to resolve it. The third listen is very important. The optician needs to listen and derive meaning to try several ideas as there is no defined guideline. The success may be achieved by embracing trial and error method. There is no single magic solution for an unfamiliar problem. There are no rules as well, as we try to accomplish something. The goal is to find out the patient satisfaction. Sometimes it takes a leap of insight. Either you hit on it or you do not. Those who hit have the WOW moment and those who do not have the AHA moment. It is like untangling the cords behind a desk. You also need to learn the art of drawing a line. When I deal with my complaining patient, I involve them in the process of management by talking to them in a very positive and friendly manner and that is how I almost always get unparallel cooperation from them. Many times they only lead me to find out the appropriate solution.

BIBLIOGRAPHY

1. Fannin TE, Grosvenor T. Clinical Optics. Butterworth Publishers; 1987.
2. Obsfeld H. Spectacle Frame and Their Dispensing.
3. Brooks CW, Borish IM. System for Ophthalmic Dispensing. Professional Press, Inc. 1979.
4. Bhootra AK. Ophthalmic Lenses. 1st ed. 2009.
5. Bhootra AK. Optician's Guide. 2nd ed. 2010.
6. Wakefield KG. Bennett's Ophthalmic Prescription Work. 3rd ed. 1994.
7. Sasieni LS. Spectacle Fitting and Optical Dispensing. 1950.
8. Topliss WS. Optical Dispensing and Workshop Practice.
9. Jalie M. Ophthalmic Lenses and Dispensing. 2nd ed. 2003.
10. Duke-Elder S, Abrams D. System of Ophthalmology—Ophthalmic Optics and Refraction.1970; 5.
11. Meister D, Sheedy JE. Introduction to Ophthalmic Optics. Carl Zeiss Vision.
12. Ophthalmic Spectacle Frame Materials, Continuing Education Course, Approved by the American Board of Opticianry.
13. Walsh G. The Product We Rely on—Part 2, Spectacle Frame Materials.
14. Ophthalmic Lens Files, By Essilor International. 1997.
15. Griffiths G. Colour Preference—a Comparative Study.
16. Jalie M. Materials for Spectacle Lenses.
17. Fowler C. Dispensing VI: Spectacle Lens Design—New and Future.
18. Cook PR. Using MRPs to Optimize Lens Performance.
19. Carr D. Selecting, Filling and Fitting Wrap Prescription Eyewear.
20. RC Palmer. KBco Wrap Solutions™— Lab Reference Manual ©.
21. Meister D. High-Powered Lenses and Thickness.
22. Disanto M. Base Curve Basics.
23. Walker P. The Truth about Base Curve.11
24. Heiting G, Shupnick MM. Progressive Lenses Replace Bifocals for Age-Defying Appearance.

25. Pierce LL. Demystifying Full Back—Surface (FBS) Progressive Lens Design.

26. Meister DJ. Progress in the Spectacle Correction of Presbyopia, Part 1: Design and Development of Progressive Lenses.

27. Meister DJ. Progress in the Spectacle Correction of Presbyopia, Part 2: Modern Progressive Lens Technologies.

28. Fine, Hoffman, Sims. Getting Used to Bifocals.

29. Mesiter D. Lens Marking Guidelines, Issued by The Vision Council, Version 2010 March 1.0.

30. University V. A Guide to the Successful Fitting of Varilux Lenses, Published.

31. Meister D. Optics of Progressive Lenses.

32. Pope DR. Progressive Addition Lenses: History, Design, Wearer Satisfaction and Trends.

33. Chapman P. Prism Doesn't Have to Be Perplexing.

34. Jalie M. Materials for Spectacle Lenses.

35. Occupational Dispensing, A Reference Guide to Professional Advice and Solutions for Workplace. Associations of British Dispensing Opticians.

36. Karp A. Dispensing Goes Digital, New Measuring Technologies Enhance Precision and Personalization Techniques.

37. Essilor's Visioffice Manual.

38. Rodenstock Impressionist 3 Manual.

39. The Rimless Eyewear Handbook. A Publication of The Rimless Eyewear Council.

40. www.laramyk.com/resources/education/dispensing.

41. www.harisingh.com/OpticalCourse.htm.

INDEX

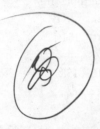

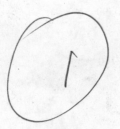